IT'S NOT (JUST)
ABOUT
—— the ——
BREAST

The Cancer Road Less Walked
A Young Woman's Cancer Story

PETRINA BURNETT

First published by Ultimate World Publishing 2021
Copyright © 2021 Petrina Burnett

ISBN

Paperback: 978-1-922497-84-0
Ebook: 978-1-922497-85-7

Cover design: Ultimate World Publishing
Layout and typesetting: Ultimate World Publishing
Editor: Rebecca Low
Cover Image: © West Australian Newspapers Limited

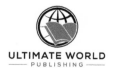

Ultimate World Publishing
Diamond Creek,
Victoria Australia 3089
www.writeabook.com.au

Testimonials

•————————————————•

In this account of the impact of breast cancer and living with an inherited cancer predisposition gene as a young woman, Petrina has managed to convey not only her personal challenges, courage and triumphs, but also articulated many of the challenges, heartaches, hurdles and opportunities facing all young women diagnosed either with cancer at an early age or with a genetic susceptibility to cancer.

I believe this book will be an inspiration for many women and their families who must face these issues. It provides invaluable advice on how this one remarkable woman overcame many of her personal hurdles to not just survive, but to live, thrive and kick ass!

Prof. Christobel Saunders, Order of Australia, FRACS.
Professor Surgical Oncology
University of Western Australia

Petrina Burnett's book is a must-read for young women affected by breast cancer, BRCA mutation carriers, and women at high risk of breast and ovarian cancer, as well as their partners, families and friends. The book is a moving and deeply human account of the confronting experiences and choices faced by a young breast cancer survivor.

Petrina recounts her 14-year cancer journey with honesty, dignity and compassion and beautifully demonstrates how resilience can help us move towards a better tomorrow. Petrina's book will give hope to young women who follow her path and shows that it is possible to live a full and rewarding life after cancer.

Assoc. Prof. Paul Cohen, FRANZCOG, MD.
Director Gynaecological Cancer Research, St John
of God Hospital, Subiaco, Western Australia

I felt hope, strength and sadness, but most of all pride throughout reading this book. Not only does it show the power of one woman's experience about life, love and the impact of breast cancer for the young woman, but it also tells of Petrina's extraordinary life and how she has utilised her skills to empathise, listen, research and understand the needs of voiceless.

Petrina's reflections are a true insight, showing that the impacts of breast cancer not only affect the individual, but also the entire family and wider community.

Ms. Kirsten Pilatti, CEO, Breast Cancer Network
Australia

Dedication

—————•—————

To my dearest Lee Jackson, Mum, Dad, Ebi and family.

And to the women who came before me and to all who have helped and inspired me along the way.

"Live as if you were to die tomorrow.
Learn as if you were to live forever."
—Mahatma Gandhi

Contents

Introduction

•————————————————————————•

Over the recent years, I have felt compelled to write about my breast cancer experience as a young woman who carries a high cancer risk susceptibility gene called BRCA1. Breast cancer is less common and sometimes misunderstood when diagnosed in this less resilient life phase, therefore proving to be a more difficult and isolating experience than what might meet the eye. Many unique challenges can arise, particularly socially, financially, psychologically and professionally. So rather than just talk about my breast cancer and preventative ovarian cancer treatment, I have wanted to focus more on these broader impacts of my cancer diagnosis, and how both myself and others have navigated and/ or resolved them.

Another objective I've had in writing this book, has been to share my family's story about our inherited BRCA1 genetic cancer mutation, hoping it may add a depth of understanding about genetic diseases, its intergenerational complexities and losses, and the impacts that it can bring from the past, through the present and into the future.

I hope that our story may give you hope and strength to make your tomorrow even better than your today, even if you're tired or it feels hard to do. I also hope that you find our learnings and insights helpful and thought-provoking, and that they remove feelings of isolation and provide clarity.

Please remember that every person's cancer story is unique, and medical practices are always progressing, so the information provided in this book may not be applicable to either your own or other people's cancer experiences or journeys. If reading this book brings up any questions or concerns relating to cancer care, I urge you to consult your treating oncology team, medical practitioner, local cancer organizations, or the appropriate organization(s) listed in the back of this book.

Happy reading and be well, strong and courageous. Petrina x

It's Not (Just) About the Breast
Find us at:
www.wellstrongcourage.com
breastbook@wellstrongcourage.com

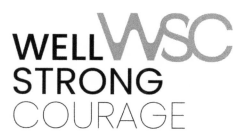

MY STORY

The Beginning and the Past.

———•———

1.

My Cancer Diagnosis. Just The Beginning.

———————————•———————————

"Virescit Vulnere Virtus -
Courage Grows Strong at the Wound"
—Burnett Clan Motto

So much can end up being in a name, or at least that is what I have come to discover over the past 14 years or so. The motto *"Virescit Vulnere Virtus"* or "Courage grows strong at the wound" was awarded to the Burnett Clan by Mary Queen of Scots, no doubt due to their gallant efforts displayed during many bloody battles of Scotland in times gone by. However, centuries later, my family would see courage growing stronger from wounds quite different than those sustained in warfare of the past. We would experience our own individual wounds from breast and ovarian cancer, generation after generation, interlinked, but nevertheless framed by the contexts of the changing medical care and technologies around each one of us, at each point in time. Our wounds would stretch beyond just the physical, with some easily seen and understood, to others being more invisible, misconceived and even isolating. Our battle would eventually be found in the mystery of our imperfect DNA, and our courage would be to outsmart it.

My first consciousness of cancer genetics was whilst working as a physiotherapist in the late 90s. I had been keeping in touch with the genetics medical literature, and had seen articles emerge relating particularly to breast and ovarian cancers. After turning the 30s corner, the time around which breast cancer had reared it's head for my Aunt, Dad's sister, and knowing that I more strongly resembled the Burnett side of the family, I had raised the matter with my general practitioner. She sought advice, and was informed that the best person to undergo genetic testing was my aunt. My Aunt Merrel was in the USA at the time. Genetic testing was also very involved and given that there had only (apparently) been two cancers in the family, I decided not to pursue the testing process. However, sadly not even a year later, I would find myself becoming another family "statistic" of this ongoing life-threatening genetic story.

Finding my Armpit Lump

I discovered my cancer in February 2007 at the end of the working week. I'd gone from having a busy working day at Fremantle Hospital in Perth, Western Australia, to being relaxed on my couch watching the evening news. I was watching footage of a well-known Australian cricket commentator behaving badly in relation to the fundraising work of the now late Jane McGrath and the McGrath Foundation. The foundation was raising funds for breast cancer support at a cricket match, a cause close to Jane's heart as she confronted her metastatic breast cancer diagnosis with her young children and cricketer husband Glen by her side. The McGraths were evidently experiencing a very difficult time, so I was confused as to why this commentator would turn her suffering into some sort of flippant joke by imitating playing the violin, as though the occasion needed a sorrowful serenade or the like! Unfortunately for him, he hadn't realized that his shenanigans had been caught on camera and telecast around the entire country. However, even bad publicity can be good when it comes to health promotion. And for me, the attention that he inadvertently drew to the cause was going to be extraordinarily helpful and timely.

In the weeks prior, I'd felt a bit heavier and different in my breast and pectoral area, so given my physiotherapy-like curiosity, I decided to investigate the issue. And there it was. My finger landed straight onto a large marble-sized lump in my left armpit. I was stunned and confused, and remember thinking that this must have been a mistake as my armpit had seemed normal not so long ago. How do lumps suddenly appear? I thought.

Eventually despite my bewilderment, my mind calmed and rational logic stepped in.

As luck had it, my sister knew of a fabulous general practitioner (GP) rostered to work the next morning called Linley. I was very grateful to find such a knowledgeable, skilled and proactive practitioner. Linley too was concerned about the history of cancer on Dad's side of the family, even though my other risk factors of breast cancer were virtually negligible. She performed a breast and armpit examination, also finding an adjacent breast lump to my armpit lump. She therefore didn't hesitate to refer me for diagnostic imaging via a mammogram, ultrasound and fine-needle aspiration, first thing the following Monday morning. By the following Thursday, the fine needle aspiration results had determined that I had a high-grade breast malignancy.

Having been on the other side of healthcare as a physiotherapist for some ten years already, I knew beyond question that my first real interaction as a patient with the health system was going to be an involved, less common and complex one. Some of my circumstances weren't great, either. I was 31 years old, the sole breadwinner, living alone and working in a particularly breast cancer treatment "unfriendly job" as I had been undertaking demanding work as a hospital physiotherapist. I was also quite nervous because I knew I didn't have a typical breast cancer presentation with more tumour in my armpit than my breast, but given that Linley was behind me one hundred percent and given that my aunt had survived her breast cancer, my confidence was lifted. By Thursday, again thanks to Linley's exemplary ability to advocate and manage my care, I was sitting in my breast surgeon's room to discuss the plan going forward.

My First Breast Surgery

My surgeon David was a very caring and empathetic man who proved to be a guiding light, ably steering the ship of my initial breast cancer treatment pathway. Breast oncology was clearly much more than just a job for him. David said that I would initially be spared the mastectomy as my breast MRI hadn't shown any other cancers in either my left or right breast. This gave me some relief as it was one less thing to deal with for the time being. However, due to having enlarged metastatic cancer deposits in my armpit or axillary lymph nodes, he said that my nodes would have to be removed outright as sentinel node biopsy sampling wasn't going to tell us any more than we already knew. So, I went on to have breast-conserving surgery and axillary clearance, removing level 1 and 2 lymph nodes a few days after my initial consultation.

Going into the appointment with David, I had thought that my chance of breast cancer survival was going to be quite good, even though I seemed to have more armpit involvement than most. I'd heard at the time that the odds of early breast cancer survival at five years was about 90%, so these statistics, combined with all the pluses that I'd entered the diagnosis with, such as being young, fit, healthy and otherwise well, made me think that I'd be ok. However, in my naivety, being greener to the cancer world from a knowledge-based point of view, I hadn't thought much about individual prognoses potentially being so varied. I discovered there are many pathological, histological and biological characteristics between the different subtypes of breast cancer, hence I then came to realise that the range of potential cancer recurrence risks and survival prognoses can vary from one person to the next quite considerably.

The tumour I had was a locally advanced grade 3 invasive intraductal basal type triple-negative breast cancer (negative of oestrogen, progesterone, and Her2 receptors), responsible for only 10-15% of all breast cancers. This tumour was a faster-growing one than most and offered no specific targeted treatment, but rather options of just surgery, chemotherapy and radiation therapy. This lack of targeted treatment offered to women with other breast cancers such as hormone receptor-positive and Her2 positive subtypes, alongside the triple negative's more aggressive "behaviour", unfortunately also typically came with a lower survival rate. So, I had work to do and more intensive treatments to face to try and turn it around.

My Post-Treatment Care Surprises

My recovery after my breast surgeries was not what I had been expecting. I had developed a seroma, a fluid collection between my rib cage and chest, which appeared not long after my drain was removed a few days after surgery. I had no idea what it was or what I needed to do about it, but since it was sitting so high under my armpit, it wasn't particularly comfortable. Thankfully, after three weekly needle aspirations, the fluid leakage finally resolved. I then went on to develop cording, consisting of the formation of a few long, tender tight bands of scar tissue running from my armpit down to my elbow. The cording impeded my ability to move my arm beyond shoulder height, but thankfully given that it had only affected my left arm, I had still been able to cook and manage small jobs around the home. Breast physiotherapy was still in it's infancy, so given that specialist treatment was limited (except for lymphoedema or swelling management), I put my good generalist physiotherapy skills to the test and thankfully managed to treat the cording successfully. I gained near to full movement of my arm by about five to six weeks post-op, just in time to be able to go back to work and drive, as advised.

Radiology Concerns

After surgery, David referred me for a string of investigations, including a CT and bone scan. There was one hairy moment after surgery that had us sitting on the edge of our seats following the CT and the bone scan. My radiologists had found an aberration in my left ribcage not far from where my breast cancer had been. As this baseline scan was needed to rule out whether I had de novo metastatic or advanced cancer at initial diagnosis, this rib issue was of concern. The radiologists were reportedly "scratching their heads" about the finding, but thankfully, they soon diagnosed a fibrodysplasia, where fibrous tissue had abnormally formed in my rib rather than bone. So, all was well for me with no visible signs of metastatic deposits, hence we now knew that we were dealing with a diagnosis of early breast cancer. However, the question still remained whether some microscopic deposits were lurking in the background, undetectable to the eye on CT and bone scan. This would be the space where the chemotherapy and radiation would now have to work within, to further increase my chances of survival.

The Breast Cancer Network Australia

After surgery, but before starting chemotherapy, I was lucky enough to connect with the Breast Cancer Network Australia (BCNA). Through their national consumer education activities and services, I started my cancer journey well informed and supported, particularly surrounding issues regarding breast cancer in young women, breast MRIs and managing chemotherapy treatment. The Founder and CEO, Lynn Swinburne, and her team, including my wonderful cousin Kirsten, had worked hard by lobbying the government, collaborating with state and federal peak cancer bodies, and growing the organization to service its 25,000 members in just nine years after it's establishment.

The Perth forum was very helpful, especially being able to hear other women talk about their personal experiences with breast cancer. It gave me both strength and inspiration to move through the cancer pathway and linked me into a larger network of women across the country who had already been there and done that. It was so important for me to connect with others, given that Perth was the most isolated city in the world and particularly also, as social media platforms like Facebook were barely in use at that time. One thing that I did soon notice in the breast cancer space however, was that I was one of the few very young women diagnosed with breast cancer.

We were a rarer find with only about 26 women being diagnosed with breast cancer under the age of 35 in Western Australia in 2007. So at the time of going through breast cancer treatment, although I'd met others who had some parallels to my emerging experience, I didn't have the opportunity to have treatment alongside anyone who was of a similar age, in a similar situation (single, without children and a possible gene mutation carrier) and in the same state. So my experience would still prove to be somewhat isolating for some time, even though from the outside, it could look like I was amongst a sea of breast cancer.

Chemotherapy

About a month after my breast and lymph node surgery, I attended my first appointment with my medical oncologist, Arlene. Arlene was a woman big in knowledge, skill and personality, but contrastingly small in stature. You could see her smallness, but feel her greatness through her presence, power, passion and positive energy. Arlene was keen to start chemotherapy the day following my first consultation, but given that I'd just found out what was in store for me, I opted to start the following week to build and ready my psychological and emotional strength. I felt vulnerable not knowing how my body would cope with this gamut of treatment. As far as drugs had been concerned, I'd only had the odd Panadol here and there, so I knew that chemotherapy would be a huge adjustment for my previously unscathed and nurtured body. Having chemo wasn't a decision that I needed to make, as the pros in my situation far outweighed the cons. Knowing that the cancer had already significantly metastasized to my armpit, the chances that it had started to make a home elsewhere in my body was high. Chemo was after all, there to do its job to increase my chances of a cure, all things willing, hopefully for another 60 years or so.

I started a fairly new regime in the world of breast cancer called dose-dense chemotherapy, given over four months rather than the more traditional six-month period. I had four cycles of two drugs called Adriamycin and Cyclophosphamide (AC) and four cycles with Paclitaxel (T) every two weeks. The immediate side effects weren't particularly nice, but I saw the nausea, vomiting, hair loss, etc., as short-term effects that were more uncomfortable and superficial by nature, and not so fundamental. I would soon discover, however, that I would have bigger fish to fry, with medium and longer-term chemotherapy side effects being more confronting and difficult, particularly for the younger woman. However, in the meantime as I undertook chemotherapy treatment, I found that absorbing some of Arlene's effervescence would prove to be medicine in itself. She certainly gave me a positive mindset and the confidence I needed to get through.

I would think that seeing a daughter go through breast cancer and chemotherapy would make any mother feel like it should have been her, and I know that Mum had to reconcile this notion often. Mum wanted to take away the pain, but the only thing she could do to help would be to listen, and to remain present and supportive as much as possible throughout the treatment pathway. Mum was also double my age at 61, the average age that women are usually diagnosed with breast cancer. Just before I started chemo, when our stress was at its highest, I recall that Mum had been keen that I purchase a wig. Deep down, I think the proposition of losing my hair was just another sign for those around me including Mum, that I really was a cancer patient and would soon go from being otherwise well to being unwell from chemo.

So, one day, Mum gently suggested that we go wig shopping! I much preferred the option of scarves, hats, or the bald look, so I responded by saying something laconic, along the lines that I wished she'd just lay off this wig thing! Mum responded saying, *"I didn't know I was laying on!"* I was glad that humour entered the piece early as it was so much easier to cope when the pressure was on and the going got tough. It also taught me earlier, that we needed to see things for what they were and to respect each other for our generational and personal differences as we began to negotiate my pathway. My niece Ruby also had to be educated on what I was about to confront, including my impending hair loss. She had turned three, and Alice and Ashleigh, my other nieces, were one. Upon starting chemo, my sister had told Ruby that I'd soon be losing my hair for a little while to help me get all better again. "Just like the bald man?" Ruby asked, referring to their neighbour across the road who had a shaved head. She'd certainly got the visuals right, and like many children I came across, wasn't at all phased seeing my bald head look.

Ruby and my other nieces would also prove to be a delight and were a beautiful antidote to the ugliness of the chemo space around me at the time. I loved seeing their joy, good health, and growth and development, to remind myself that there was still beauty and good out there. Their youth and vitality were like medicine, as was seeing that life held so much promise for them.

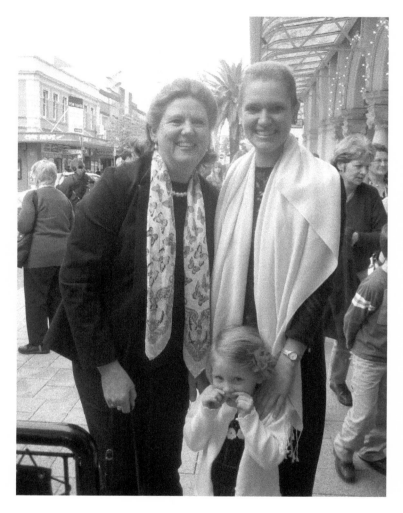

Ruby, Mum and I at the theatre.

During this time of more intensive treatments, my family and friends did many things for me, big and small. Their gestures and kindness spoke very loudly and made my recovery so much easier. They would ring and drop in often to check up on me, cook nutritious immune-boosting food and broths, take me out for meals (when I wasn't nauseous) and make sure that I was going ok mentally and emotionally.

On the physical front chemo-wise, I dropped to about 53 kgs on AC chemo (which was on the low side for my height) as I'd lost my appetite due to my nausea not being the best. The fifth in-line anti-nausea medication called lorazepam, was the only one that got my nausea levels to where they needed to be, but given it's strong sedative effect, I often avoided taking it, given that I was working during treatment (I also understand that anti-nausea medication has continued to improve since 2007). But thankfully, after a couple of months, the nausea ceased when I started Paclitaxel. On the Paclitaxel, the side effects were more tolerable and my weight normalised. I did, however, then need to contend with some new arthritic like aches and pains in my back and hips, making me feel like I'd strangely gone from being 31 to 91 in a very short span of time. Thankfully, simple things helped to alleviate my geriatric-like discomforts, including warmth, movement and gentle exercise. It made me realise how it could sometimes be the simple and free things in life that could help the most.

Before I finished my last chemotherapy cycle, I bought a beautiful dog called Ebi (short for Ebony). Ebi was a small, exuberant, energetic and affectionate smooth-haired fox terrier. She was keen and enthusiastic, gutsy and tender, and was always in for the fun of it. She looked out for me in an almost intuitive way during these changing times and gave me never-ending companionship and TLC. She mitigated some of the destabilization and heaviness that cancer had brought to my world, and gave my life a purpose for the coming years, in a way that was therapeutic and needed.

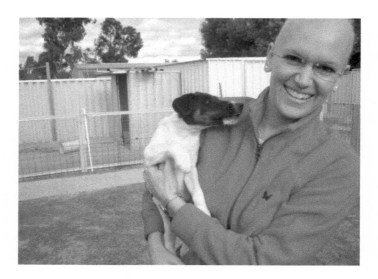

Ebi and I.

As the chemo phase came to an end, it was certainly a relief. After a month's reprieve, however, I would soon again be swept up with ongoing treatment with the commencement of radiation therapy.

2.

Moving Through Treatment. Early Survival.

"Hope is being able to see there is light despite...the darkness.."
—Desmond Tutu

Radiation and the End of 2007

A month or so after chemotherapy ended saw me enter the sphere of radiotherapy with Mandy. Mandy, my radiation oncologist, had a real knack for connecting with me as a younger person, and consequently came to be one of my favourite treating doctors. I knew that she really understood me, the challenges I'd had, and what I had in front of me. Mandy knew I had been thinking of dodging the radiation bullet as I had the bilateral mastectomies seed planted due to my family cancer history, but her convincing comment of, *"oh well, I'll still be radiating into your armpit and above your collarbone,"* sold it to me quite frankly. The 9% improved survival benefit with radiotherapy was also a bit too high to just walk away from.

The six weeks of daily radiation treatments, including five days of boost therapy, flew by. My hair had just started to regrow, forming a chic style that was really quite nice for a change. And of course, there were no bad hair days! The treatments gave my day structure, having paused on the work front to give myself a break after chemo. I moved through radiation with relative ease, only experiencing a minor skin reaction in the short-term and some breast lymphoedema or swelling for the medium-term. Thankfully, the breast oedema settled after six months or so, which was great because my breast heaviness made returning to exercise more difficult. I often had to manually hold my left breast when jogging, as even good bras couldn't hold it adequately upon impact!

Unlike during my chemotherapy phase of care, during radiation, I was able to live the cancer experience alongside a lovely couple who lived in Perth. Cam, like me, was being looked after by Mandy. Cam had initially been diagnosed with a type of leukaemia called plasmacytoma, but unfortunately his diagnosis progressed into multiple myeloma within months of meeting him. By a stroke of fate, I'd also met his wife Libby as we had both been working for the Metropolitan Area Health Service collaborating on a chronic disease program a month or so prior. We walked the path of cancer together, removing quite a bit of the isolation, sharing notes, keeping each other company and just getting on with where life was taking us. Our relationship was so valuable, being like-minded, having similar values and interests and being of similar age. I found that living the cancer experience in the same phase of care together in real-time could really help you move through, and the friendships formed could become so meaningful, helpful and special.

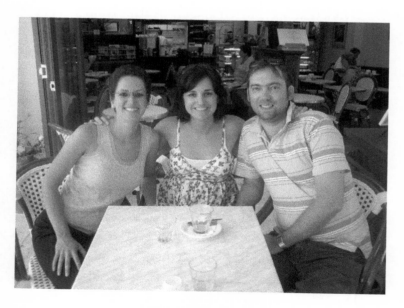

Cam, Libby and I

After Treatment Prognosis and Reflections

Once my "active treatment" phase finished at the end of radiation in late September, I ended up having all that cancer medicine could offer to treat my breast cancer, and it was now up to me and my body alone to get me through. I only asked then what my survival odds would be. *"A bit better than 50%,"* was Mandy's response, way off the 90% five year survival rate that I'd come to know. How close my survival odds were to 60% I still don't know (and thankfully don't need to), but I got the message. Although my prognosis could have been worse as I know it can be for others, it still felt like a blow after enduring all those treatments and after all the hard work that both myself and my treating team had put in.

I still remained positive that I would survive, given that my aunt had and given that I'd received the best and latest care possible. However, I would still have times when I'd lose my nerve upon the emergence of metastatic disease-like symptoms such as pain, where I'd think, *"oh my goodness, is this the beginning of the end?"* Naturally, I could not and did not want to get my head around the possibility of not making it. I had thought that if I was to pass, my life would have seemed to have been about so little, not having done much or achieved much as yet. By some stroke of luck, the foundation of my thinking seemed to always tip back toward the notion that I'd be ok, even though I would have contrasting moments where I realised that this might just be wishful thinking.

What might have helped give me confidence also was that I'd had faith in, and had really appreciated, my relationship with my treating team. There had also been a healthy respect and acknowledgement of my background in healthcare. They also hadn't shown any concern at all with me calling them by their first names. But in all honesty, I found first name terms were more natural, gave me more of a sense of control as a patient, and also kept me in my normal sphere as a colleague. In some way too, I'd also come to find my conversations with them of some comfort and a space where I felt more understood than I had felt in the outside world. I was a patient but wasn't fully one either. This space I came to call "no man's land."

Early Survivorship

After I finished treatment, I went across to Melbourne to attend a National Young Women's Breast Cancer Forum. It was wonderful as I met more women who shared a similar experience to me, including more BRCA1 mutation carriers, the mutation that my doctors suspected that I had. One of the women that I met was called Jude. Jude was diagnosed at 24 years of age around 2006 with two different types of breast cancer, one in her left breast, the other in her right. She was originally from the country in Western Australia (WA) and had gone through the same school as me, some five or so years later. Although our contact was limited by living in different states and time zones, Jude was my shining beacon and someone I could chat to about breast and genetic stuff. She'd had a pretty tough time with her cancer by all accounts, but I always enjoyed seeing the smile on her face and her zest for life.

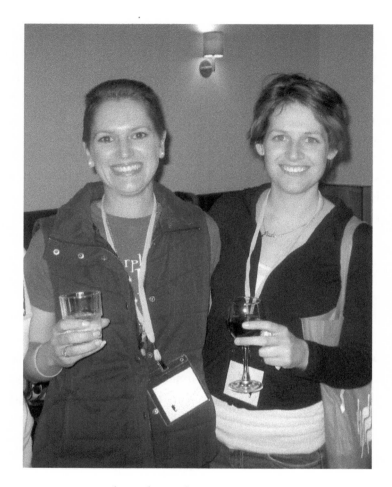

**Jude and I at the young women's
symposium in Melbourne**

I also really cherished my friendships outside of the cancer
space. Although some of my friends may have been less aware of
what I was going through, I found that catching up with them
helped me to realign the imbalance that the cancer world could
sometimes bring. The contrasting wellness and normality of

their world were also enticing to be immersed in, and personally helped me regain a broader perspective on the world outside that my cancer experiences and treatments had made more insular and narrow. I also realised that relationships with my friends, old and new, had been so important to help me get through and stay on track during this time, and it was especially in times like this that I realized that my friends and family loved me a lot, and would be there, in good times and bad. I was so grateful to have their endless and steadfast support.

Besides keeping in touch with friends and getting back to work after radiation, I also found some comfort in this earlier phase by getting back to my exercise. It helped keep my positivity and spirits up about my prognosis, particularly now as my body was left to its own devices given that my cancer had no existing targeted treatment options, being a triple negative cancer. I found that a formal exercise program gave me a sense that I was still having ongoing treatment, improving my survival odds and moving towards wellness and recovery. It also helped me ward off my intermittent feelings of "survival dissonance" that all of us go through, wondering if the treatment has been enough to get us over the line.

When I started exercising again, I discovered that I'd become markedly deconditioned. When on an exercise bike especially, I noted that I'd been peddling slowly, feeling no shortness of breath or exertion, but realising that my heart rate was incredibly high. My body certainly felt foreign. I continued walking Ebi as I'd done throughout treatment and resumed swimming and gym-based exercise as my energy levels had somewhat improved. Getting moving again felt so incredibly empowering, helping me feel as though I was more in control of my body and getting me back to wellness again. Exercise would prove to be such a powerful avenue for recovery and overall healing, and would tide me over so incredibly well into my strange new world.

BRCA1 Genetic Testing

The end of 2007 would also see me have genetic testing. In 1995, Western Australia's Familial Cancer Genetic Services opened its doors for BRCA1 testing, offering a huge leap forward in the management of genetic cancers. The classic family presentation with the BRCA1 mutation saw a number of women on the same side of the family present with "triple-negative" breast cancer before the age of 40 and/or be diagnosed with high grade serous ovarian cancer before the age of 70 (EVIQ, 2019). The BRCA1 gene mutation had been discovered in 1994 by Mary-Claire King and her research team. BRCA1 (known as **BR**east **CA**ncer gene one) was an autosomal dominant genetic mutation, meaning that there was a 50% risk of inheriting it if a parent was a carrier. It didn't matter if you were male or female as both sexes carry the gene, however with this specific mutation, women carried the main burden of risk. Men can carry and pass on the mutation also, but do not personally present with ovarian cancer of course, nor appear to present with breast cancer as women do.

So in October, after chemotherapy and after completing all the necessary paperwork (including locating my grandmother's death certificate and getting my aunt's consent to the release of her medical records), I set off to King Edward Memorial Hospital in Perth to have the genetic counselling and blood tests. During the consultation, I was told that it could be a wait of up to 18 months to get my results back due to the waitlist and the technological capacity, but at least by the end of the year, the testing process was in motion. It was time for a break now anyhow, and that I would have through my summer holiday with family, friends and Ebi in the South West of WA.

Conclusion

My diagnosis and treatment had already been quite a ride of its own. However, in my heart of hearts, I had an inkling that despite all I'd already gone through, I was going to have many more hurdles ahead of me and have to endure times much harder. For now though, the new year reprieve would be a time to gather strength, have a good time, and work on returning to wellness and empowerment.

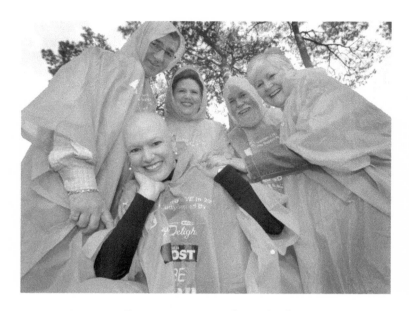

Mum, Dad, our cousins Jude and Alan, and I.
© West Australian Newspapers Limited.

3.

The Genetic Past And The Now Changeable Future.

"In every conceivable manner, the family is a link to our past, bridge to our future."

—Alex Hale

The genetic testing process that I entered in late 2007, would prove to be a lifesaver but would also prove to bring more complexity with it. Not only would both myself and potentially my brother and sister now need to manage further cancer risks, but like any woman at 32, although I wanted to keep my breasts and ovaries to see me through, the challenge would be that keeping them also came with the risk of developing further cancers. How long I could safely hold out for, no one could say for certain either. And although the concept to just move on with my life and put cancer all behind me was nice, I knew that for me personally and as a family, we still had many hoops to jump through first.

My BRCA1 Genetic Results

Four months after my genetic testing in January 2008, Genetic Services called to make an appointment with my clinical geneticist. Jenny informed me that I had inherited the BRCA1 gene mutation. My family's gene mutation involved a deletion on our 17th chromosome's DNA sequence, which controls and regulates the suppression of tumours. When tumour suppressor genes are functional, they are normal genes that slow down cell division, repair DNA mistakes and tell cells when to die (a process that is known as apoptosis or programmed cell death) (American Cancer Society, 2020). In light of our specific family history and my individual case, it was predicted that I still ran a 60% risk of developing another new primary breast cancer and a 60% risk of developing ovarian, peritoneal, or fallopian tube cancer over my lifetime. I was also told that some other cancer risks might also be slightly increased, but to the best of their knowledge at that point in time, breast and ovarian cancers were the obvious players in the BRCA1 space.

My genetic counsellor asked me how I felt about the confirmed genetic diagnosis. I don't recall saying much as I knew that anything I might have tried to say would have sounded inept and trite. We clearly now had confirmation that our reality would soon be even more complicated, particularly as the news spread across my immediate and wider family. My thoughts around the diagnosis were already conflicting and multi-layered, and as of yet, the consequences were academic and had not been lived through. They were rather made up of isolated facts, pockets of memories and patchy information. I used to joke that the notion of starting from square one again and trading in my DNA was the best option, but as with any adversity, we are given our lot in life, and our job is to just deal with it in the best way we can. I would soon find out too, that the consequences of carrying the gene mutation would be big not only from a physical, emotional and social perspective, but also a legal one. Since the advent of genetic testing and the identification of genetic flaws and mutations, increasing insurance policy discrimination had emerged, making it more difficult for us to get insurance, such as income protection and life insurance. Travel insurance after a cancer diagnosis also proved to be more difficult to obtain.

The big plus with the confirmed BRCA1 gene mutation diagnosis of course was that the scientific knowledge that came with it could positively influence my and our survival going forward. It was recommended at the very least, that I have ongoing breast and ovarian screening (the latter was recommended at the time, but not currently). It was also recommended that I consider having preventative surgeries by removing my breasts and ovaries. In terms of my ovaries, I wanted to keep my sex hormones like oestrogen, and remain pre-menopausal for as long as I could. So many organs and tissues of the body would otherwise be affected, including my heart, brain and bone health. I also still had the hope of pregnancy, so in my mind, I wanted to keep my ovaries intact at least for the rest of the decade, to try and make my hopes a reality. I was also happy holding onto my breasts for the time being as I liked my body and didn't like the option of either needing a part of me to be man-made, or having to wear removable breast prostheses.

So, I was stuck in a place of dissonance between a rock and a hard place, not liking the look of either screening or surgical options, but knowing I was on borrowed time. Screening was only more likely to pick up cancers earlier than might have been the case otherwise. They didn't prevent cancers from happening of course. So the way that I saw it, screening would really just be an option to hold the fort up for the time being, until I was ready for preventative or prophylactic surgery, until a suspicious lesion cropped up on imaging, and/ or until I lost my nerve.

Before I made any moves with my own BRCA1 management, I decided to get my head around the past, as in some way, I knew it would help me to deal with the present, and be able to plan for the future. So I looked a little further into our ancestry, searching for any suspicious signs of breast or ovarian cancer on my paternal side of the family. I knew that this wasn't going to be straight forward beyond my grandmother's passing, as there had been no cancer registry in existence. Death certificates were also very hit and miss, tending to cite the actual signs and symptoms causing death rather than the conditions or diagnoses driving it. So we decided to look more for medical signs of metastatic cancer, such as the typical lung, liver and brain metastases found in the cancers of BRCA1 mutation carriers, and we discovered some interesting, but naturally sad findings.

My Great-Great-Grandmother, Charlotte

My great-great-grandmother, Charlotte Weaver, was the first ancestor who appeared to have succumbed to a BRCA1 related death in 1914 at the age of 46. Charlotte was the daughter of a convict. Just 15 months before her death, she appeared on the inaugural Register of Midwives in Western Australia, having gained much respect and admiration for her work as a Perth based midwife. It seems likely that she passed from disseminated metastatic breast or ovarian cancer to her lungs and liver, having *"ascites, cirrhosis, pneumonia and operation"* listed as the causes of death on her death certificate. Presumably, her symptoms were of concern to her physicians at what is now called Royal Perth Hospital, hence explaining why she was taken to the operating theatre to investigate the issue. It would be likely that upon seeing signs of her extensive lung and liver metastases, that her surgeons knew that it would not be possible to intervene and save her. Of note also, is that fact that two of her sisters also passed in their earlier 30s and mid 50s, with suspicious BRCA1 cancer related symptoms. However, without clear surgical or DNA evidence, it's not possible to confirm these either way.

My Grandmother Charlotte

My paternal grandmother, Charlotte Burnett, appears to be the next to be affected by the gene mutation back in 1976. Her father, James Weaver (the late Charlotte Weaver's son), was likely to be the BRCA1 mutation carrier. My grandmother was 56 and for some time, had been complaining about symptoms like abdominal bloating and lethargy, only to be told by doctors that there was nothing wrong with her and that her issues were rather psychosomatic or in her head. It would soon be very clear however, that a serious medical issue was at hand. Upon undertaking investigative surgery, my grandmother was diagnosed with stage 4 ovarian cancer, whereby her cancer had extended profusely through her bowel and liver. After her extensive gynae-debulking surgery, her medical team knew they were clutching at straws.

As chemotherapy had not yet been in routine use for ovarian cancer, my grandma's doctors trialled a very experimental treatment delivered by the Tronado machine. It was a last-ditch effort whereby the microwave treatment attempted to slow the cancer down in its tracks. However, this reportedly did more harm than good. Sadly, my gran only lived for another six months after her initial diagnosis, and by all accounts, it was a very poor quality six months with multiple bowel obstructions, a lot of discomfort and little dignity. I can only imagine how awful an experience it must have been for everyone to see and to live through.

Living through my grandma's palliative stages came with heartache too. My grandfather formed an emotional connection with another lady, as my gran faced her end. This relationship beginning, combined with my grandfather's limited ability to articulate his emotions, contributed to and manifested unideal family dynamics for some time. Another complication also presented on a financial front. Not long prior to my grandmother's illness, a large loan had been secured to expand the family business. However not long after my grandmother's death, the family soon had a large death tax bill with little liquid cash to be able to pay it, adding yet another strain at a time that was already challenged. So the multifactorial and unexpected stresses and strains on the family would take their toll on many levels.

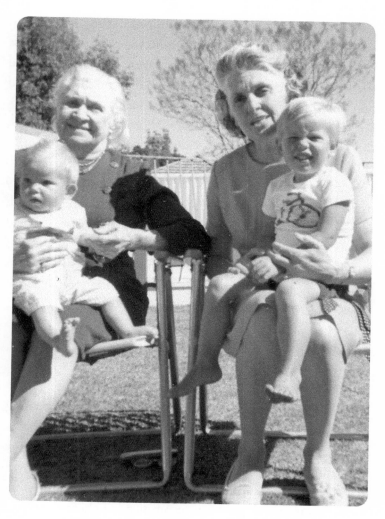

My grandmother Charlotte, great grandmother, brother Norman and sister Priscilla. We don't have any photos of my grandmother and me together, given she became unwell not long after my birth.

I was only ten months old when Grandma Charlotte died. My brother Norman was four at the time and my sister Priscilla was two. My brother was old enough to remember my parent's grief, but obviously he had little understanding of what had happened. When my BRCA1 diagnosis was confirmed all these years later, we again reflected on my grandmother's life and tried to reconcile the fact that she had died not because she'd done anything wrong (or had been stressed as some had said), but rather because she had just been born being who she was, as anyone is with a genetic disease.

Despite this reality however, on another level, there was beauty in the tragedy somehow. My siblings, cousins and I lived on with something of her in us. A few of us looked a bit like her and had developed interests that she'd had, such as music and swimming. So when we looked at the bigger picture, she was still with us through her legacy rather than her physical presence, even though we would have loved having that too.

My Aunt, Merrel

In 1984, eight years after my grandmother Charlotte's passing, my Dad's sister Merrel was diagnosed with medullary breast cancer at 34. We were shocked and saddened that cancer was happening again so soon. Merrel was a single working mum with two small children. She went on to have a mastectomy and lymph node clearance and had been recommended chemotherapy, a fairly new addition to the cancer treatment pathway at that time. I was about 9, my sister Priscilla 10, and my brother Norman 12. I remember Mum and Dad doing a lot to help Merrel, including having our cousins stay with us for the duration of her treatment. My parents kept our balls in the air as kids, and additionally looked after Gem and Tony, dropping them off at school on the other side of Perth and providing a lot of emotional and physical support. A few years later, Merrel also had some additional gynae issues, so she underwent a hysterectomy and bilateral salpingo-oophorectomies, or the removal of the uterus, ovaries and fallopian tubes on both sides. She was hence unknowingly, fortuitously spared the risk of ovarian cancer developing.

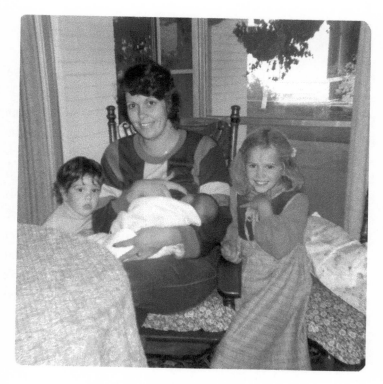

Merrel, Tony, Baby Gem and I.

This period of time was uncertain for us all, seeing my family living life again within a cancer story. My mother's father had also died from cancer before my birth in 1972, so for my family, it was our third cancer experience in 12 years and for me, a short 9 years. When my diagnosis of the BRCA1 gene mutation came through in 2008, my gran had passed 31 years prior, and Aunt Merrel had been living in the USA as a cancer survivor of 23 years. For our family and for me personally, cancer had seemingly become a way of life. It was almost normal.

The Rest of My Family

Managing the fall out of our BRCA1 diagnosis over these earlier years as a family was a sometimes messy and difficult process as I'd imagine it is for any family having to confront genetic diseases. The help that we received certainly helped us tackle managing the cancer risks themselves, but not so much beyond that. We were now all stakeholders in my, and indeed our BRCA1 diagnosis, so travelling through this post-diagnosis space would prove to bring up a complex mix of emotions. These emotions would range from sorrow to guilt, through to relief and everywhere in between. As to be expected, our individual understanding of the facts and our coping mechanisms weren't always going to be the same either, so we needed to stay connected and be patient with each other, and steer through the rough waters.

I know that Dad often felt guilty for passing on the gene, as I'm sure any parent would, but any parent shouldn't. But, what I learned was that life worked in mysterious ways. I had learned many of the very skills that I needed to cope with the fallout of my diagnosis from my parents, Dad included. These life skills would end up being incredibly helpful to manage, recover and even prosper with all that BRCA1 had brought. They showed me that hard work and tenacity were attributes that can hold you in good stead. They showed me that standing up after you've fallen over and rolling up your sleeves to get back to business has its benefits. They also showed me that resourcefulness and self-accountability were good modes to live by. So rather than feeling overwhelmed when I was diagnosed, my apparent inherited pragmatism and forward-looking stance would help me to get off to a good start.

My brother Norman and sister Priscilla had genetic testing with their results both coming back as being negative, so for my sister and my sibling's children, the risk of them developing either breast or ovarian cancer was at the normal population risk over their lifetime, not the BRCA1 risk level. We were particularly relieved that we'd been spared the anguish of my nieces potentially being mutation carriers, something that would have needed another 15 years or more to find out, as they did not qualify for testing until they could personally consent, at or after the age of 18.

When it came to medical support in this earlier phase, my sister Sil carried a lot of the load, having a background in health as a physiotherapist and also having a husband who was also a health professional. She was always very empathetic and generous of herself and her time. I know it must have been very hard for her to come to many of my appointments as a support person, particularly the more stressful ones such as my initial consultations with my breast surgeon and clinical geneticist. All the while too, she remained vulnerable to possibly carrying the BRCA1 gene mutation herself, with the added concern of having two young daughters to think about.

My brother Normie also found a way to be present during my treatment and the fall out of my cancer diagnosis. He helped me out when he could, by doing handyperson like jobs around the house, and fixing any media or IT glitches. His practical gestures meant a lot. I knew that it was probably hard to know what to say in times like this, as it would I'd imagine, for any brother.

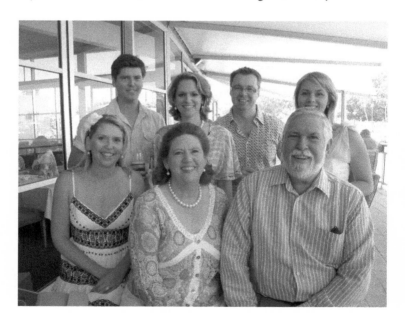

Burnett Family

Of my Dad's two brothers, one was tested and was negative, and the other avoided testing. I couldn't understand the reasons for my other uncle not being tested. It was perplexing, given that he had seen the carnage that this ongoing family story has caused. However, I understood that it can be a very personal decision for all of us and knew that either way, we all had to respect each others decisions.

In the years that followed my diagnosis, thanks to Angelina Jolie in 2013, the BRCA1 mutation arrived on the map and became more widely understood by the general public than ever before. Angelina's media work to raise awareness of genetic related cancers was very helpful for many of us. Pre-2013 when I explained to people that I had genetically related breast cancer, I'd receive some very quizzical looks as the concept was quite new and complex for the average person on the street, unless they had a medical or science background. After all, at the time of my diagnosis, the BRCA1 genetic testing procedure was only 13 years old, so community awareness and understanding were still in their infancy.

Conclusion

BRCA1 had either taken our lives, or if our lives had been spared as Merrel's and mine had been, a loss of certainty, prosperity and liberties normally attributed to young or mid-adulthood. Genetic testing, despite its tremendous privileges, also brought its complications, and with the testing and counselling process still being relatively new, we were charting the territory as we went. Within a short five years, too, we would see breast cancer present in another family member, again in a way that was heartbreaking and incredibly sad.

MY STORY

BRCA1 and
Cancer Treatment Fallout.

4.

Initial Recovery Hurdles. Reconstruction Surgery. Changes And Adversities.

_____•———————————————•_____

"Healing doesn't have to look magical or pretty. Real healing (can be) hard, exhausting...Let yourself go through it. Don't try to paint it as anything other than what it is. Be there for yourself with no judgement."

—Audrey Kitching

With aspects of my care on track for my breast cancer and BRCA1 diagnoses, I now had the job of addressing the more physical, emotional, social and psychological aspects and consequences of treatment. This involved managing my now lower energy levels, navigating work changes, and acquainting myself with what some call "the new normal." As much as I might like to sugar coat this part, I found it a struggle and in many ways, found it more confronting than the year of my actual treatment. I knew where I wanted to be, but my path would remain suspended, dealing with the longer term consequences and tangents that followed.

The Ups and Downs of Working During Treatment

The reality of the treatment and post-treatment world is that all the normal life things continue as they do for anyone else, yet you also carry the numerous superimposed health challenges that cancer brings on top of it. For me, the idea of just being able to get better in a safe and calm place away from the chaos of the workplace would have been preferable, but that was not to be, so I had to deal with both the positives and negatives of working whilst not yet being fully well. The positives were that it provided me with a support network of colleagues and brought some balance to my world. It also distracted me by making me think about others and their needs, rather than being able to overly focus on the downsides of my illness and situation. So, in many ways, I was grateful to be able to provide for myself and keep things ticking over.

Hospitals weren't appropriate places to work when having cancer treatment due to the risk of picking up infections whilst immunosuppressed, nor did recovering patients need to see a visibly unwell physio. So, I made the move to work in a non-clinical short term position, working as a project officer in chronic disease management part-time. The team that I worked with were absolutely wonderful, keeping a close eye on me and allowing me to have flexible work arrangements around my chemo sessions every two weeks. I was very lucky to have been able to work closely with a small team of exceptional people.

However, I found that working with the wider teams wasn't so smooth and added unwelcomed stress due to the existing workplace politics and culture. It was a time when anyone undergoing cancer treatment would prefer little or none. At the same time I was still managing intermittent pangs of nausea courtesy of the Adriamycin and Cyclophosphamide chemotherapy, so it wasn't going to be a walk in the park. When this position came to an end at the completion of chemotherapy I was ready to move on, however I was sad to say goodbye to the good friends and colleagues that I'd made within my immediate team. They had made me proud *"to spell my name W-O-M-A-N"* (Maya Angelou). And many of us have remained special friends, even to this day.

I had a welcomed and brief break from work during radiation, which allowed me to regroup, gain my strength and spend a bit more time exercising and recovering. However, my bank account was soon empty, so I moved into a part-time clinical physiotherapy role at Royal Perth Hospital (RPH). My work with RPH was excellent for my lower energy levels, again being more user-friendly being out of the hectic fast-paced hospital ward environment. I spent the day seeing patients requiring rehabilitation in their own homes and was thus afforded some physical downtime on the road between visits. The work environment was good and the team was lovely, so it was a happy time and was thankfully smoother sailing. However, due to undergoing my mastectomy and reconstruction surgery at the end of 2008, my employment at RPH soon came to an end.

Reconstruction Surgery

My breasts would be the first port of call after my BRCA1 diagnosis as the risk of another breast cancer in my 30s had been higher than my ovarian one. The latissimus reconstruction was the only choice that I had at that time unless I was prepared to be flat-chested and/or wear a breast prosthesis within a bra. I didn't qualify for the DIEP reconstruction as I didn't have enough fat needed for this procedure, nor did surgeons like using the abdomen as a donor site in women such as myself who hoped to childbear down the track. Additionally, subpectoral reconstructions were not recommended in my case either, as the tissues of my chest would be less durable given that I'd had chest irradiation.

The latissimus reconstruction procedure involved the relocation of the latissimus muscle to the front of my chest to form a pocket for a breast implant to rest in. The nerve supply to the muscle would be deactivated, with the pectoral muscle being divided and placed in front of the implant also. The surgery would obviously interfere with my anatomy quite significantly, but the professional consensus at the time was that these anatomical variations would have little impact on my physical function! Although I was aware of the inherent power of this muscle that attaches the spine and pelvis to the shoulder, I knew that some activities like rowing, swimming, rock climbing, doing yoga, planks, and push-ups would be affected, but to what degree, I didn't know. And although I didn't like the idea of having these physical changes with the surgery, I also did not particularly want to go from being reasonably well-breasted to flat-chested overnight. In all honesty, I had been happy with my breasts and would have loved to have not had to change them. But, I realised that I needed to focus on the cancer prevention viewpoint and the dignity I'd be getting back from the surgery, hard as that might have been for me at the time.

Being in waiting rooms was often anxiety-provoking for all sorts of reasons and would certainly make me build up a sweat. One such time this happened was when I was waiting for my first reconstruction consult. At the time, I didn't particularly enjoy sitting alongside my contemporaries who were invariably waiting for their cosmetic breast augment consultations. I was still short-haired, a bit pasty, and still hanging in there, so I found the juxtaposition uncomfortable and I felt out of place. Seeing my discomfort levels rise, my sister, Sil, would distract me with witty comments about the magazines we'd be flicking through or suggest that we pop out for a quick walk. She'd have me laughing in no time by pulling all sorts of quirky situational jokes. I loved her ability to lighten up the proceedings, despite the intense and extreme contexts that we were finding ourselves in.

My plastic and reconstructive surgeon, Tony, was a good sport and would come to see me through quite a few ups and downs over the months after my first consultation. His stellar skill, kindness and empathy helped me to continue plodding through the BRCA1 maze, and I will be forever thankful. Towards the end of my first consultation, he asked what size I would like to be after my reconstruction. Not expecting this question and being somewhat bewildered, I said that I had just wanted to be the same as I was now. *"Hmmm, that's about right,"* Tony responded as he assessed my breasts from a technical, constructional, and even artistic viewpoint. My breasts had obviously hit the bullseye for all those years, and I'd only just found out as I had them assessed to be removed. I had to laugh!

The day of my reconstruction surgery came as a shock. I woke up after the five and a half hours of surgery and momentarily thought that I'd been in a car accident and had smashed the front of my chest on the steering wheel. It felt like I had sustained a sudden significant chest injury. It was very sore. I also still had the breathing tube in my throat and was very cold and nauseous, so it was not the welcome back to consciousness I had been wanting! Thankfully however, with the recovery room staff running around like mad people, I was soon warm, experiencing no nausea, and able to speak again without the endotracheal tube in my throat. I was now back on track.

When I look back, I don't think I was consciously aware of the extent of the deeper loss that I'd had after my reconstructive surgery. Leading up to it, I had been quite mechanical in my approach, being more in my head about it's logic and processes rather than being in my heart. I now realise that I went into a state of shock for a couple of weeks after the surgery, feeling empty and foreign under my own skin in a way that is still hard to explain. I recall losing my appetite, lost more weight and actively avoided having any photos taken to avoid having any tangible memories of this early post-operative time.

The psychological changes brought on by the surgery probably weren't ones that I could have necessarily prepared for either. They were changes that I most likely needed to adjust to and recover from afterwards, given that no experience I'd had thus far was even remotely similar in nature nor magnitude. The surgery also gave me a feeling that I was again moving backward in my life rather than moving forward, which I always found a bit of a struggle. It felt like two steps forward, then one step back, and vice versa.

However, it was lovely during my hospital stay to receive many visitors, many beautiful flowers and many gifts. They reminded me that I was very loved and cared for. I also liked that my hospital room looked like a fusion of a florist shop and gift store, which removed the clinical like feel, and gave a more vibrant and wellness like feel. I really appreciated it, given that I wasn't able to leave my room for a good four days or so after surgery, as I was quite groggy and my overall mobility was initially quite impaired. Thankfully within a month or so, things started to turn around with a sort of "new me" emerging, and for that I was thankful. I managed to enjoy Christmas of 2008 a few weeks later, getting my bikinis out for a New Year's swim (or should I say paddle) with my new chest. I was naturally pleased when I discovered that my bikinis still fit! Tony had done his job well.

The short-term reconstruction expanders placed under my skin and muscle layers made my chest look like a couple of hard buns were sitting just under my skin. They were injected with saline every week for around five to six weeks, and eventually got to the size they were prior to my reconstruction. This part of the surgery was about stretching out my muscle and soft tissue layers, and was a means to an end of course, until the second surgery six months later. The second part of the surgery involved having the temporary saline expanders removed and the permanent silicon prostheses inserted. It had me looking closer to my original appearance, albeit to a point where my chest now looked a bit too good to be true.

However within about six or so months, my left nipple deviated, lifting up and out towards my armpit due to radiation fibrosis or scarring, whilst the implant also dropped as the pesky pectoral muscle had also sustained some radiation-related damage and wasn't holding the implant sufficiently. So fixing these issues took another surgical procedure (number four), but we got there thanks to Tony's amazing skill, patience and support.

Some of the changes after reconstruction were bizarre and took me a while to get used to. The implants gave a "hovercraft-like effect" when lying on my front as they didn't squash, nor did they squash to allow me to fit into various clothes as my real breasts had. My new breasts also moved as I used my pectoral and other arm muscles, so this took some time to get used to. I also now had no sensation across the front of my chest, so hugs now felt a bit feeble with the numbness. I missed the normal sensation of receiving and giving a warm wholehearted hug as I had in the past. But I still had a strong sense of dignity and a somewhat greater sense of femininity and when push comes to shove, there was much to be said for that. I realised how lucky I was compared to other women who didn't have the opportunity to have reconstruction, nor have a good "canvas" upon which to reconstruct due to their previous breast treatments. Knowing also that my family members had been worse off not so long ago also, reminded me also to be grateful to all who had contributed to getting me to where I was.

New Employment After Reconstruction

Physiotherapy wasn't a job for those when physically incapacitated, so for me, it was a juggling act to both be able to rehabilitate and pay the bills particularly after my initial breast surgery and this first reconstruction surgery. The problem with professions like physiotherapy, is that people such as myself, generally need up to two to three months to be able to return to full, or near full duties at work after these more intensive surgeries. The time is needed to physically rehabilitate and restore our arm movement and strength back to the level needed to do our jobs. It takes time for the tissues to heal. The surgery can also be quite painful, so it can take some time until movement can be restored properly without a sense of pulling or pain. It is also known that delaying the return of activity helps increase the healing outcomes of the chest, armpit and lymphatic tissue, so pacing our recovery out is very important.

With these considerations therefore, during these latissimus dorsi reconstruction surgeries I knew that I'd best move jobs again, and decided to pursue part-time physiotherapy student tutoring for two of Perth's universities. The hospital-based tutoring was perfect, particularly given my known functional limitations that would be repeating within six months at the exchange surgery. I bypassed the issue by being the brains rather than the muscle so to speak, supervising the students closely and talking them through the heavy patient handling and rehabilitation activities and procedures. I also loved being in the company of well, healthy, energized and happy young adults, as well as being back in the stimulating and busy environment of the hospital ward.

So, for those first few years in particular, my career pathway would end up being more circumstantially driven, with my employment decisions being made predominantly through need. It was as though I'd become a professional "backpacker," living from one month to the next. This was in contrast to many of my contemporaries, who were building stronger foundations, enjoying more prosperity, or even climbing the hierarchical ladder in their respective professions. Despite the professional displacement, however, I was still thankful to be able to work and have a roof over my head. I knew that some could even struggle to have that.

Physical Changes

During this first year after treatment, I'd read a little information about cancer side effects, one being that fatigue was common and that it could be a longer-term issue to contend with. I knew that the demands of my now 32-year-old work and private life, combined with my ongoing surgical treatments might contribute to a rougher ride, and I was right. Another issue was that my hormones were fluctuating terribly, having gone from being pre-menopausal prior to treatment to menopausal during it and then back to a dysfunctional and poorly regulated pre-menopausal state again after it. All of these factors led to my body systems underperforming and being sluggish, even though on assessment, my blood tests were all in the normal range. I came to realise it was the regulation and interplay collectively of these numerous biological processes that needed time to get back on track.

Unfortunately, the only direct information that I had been given about fatigue from a health provider was that a number of patients undergoing chemotherapy for breast cancer were still able to work full time! I'd remember seeing the issues that Kylie Minogue was experiencing with post-chemo fatigue, with her being carried off the stage post-performance not long after her breast cancer treatment. But how concert performing and full time working women related to my world, I just didn't know. I discovered that it was just going to be a time that I couldn't accelerate for either love or money.

My lower energy was all too clear one day, around six to nine months after I finished treatment, when I decided to ride to work to incorporate some rehabilitation back into my workday. The commute was 20 minutes along a flat cycle path each way. I'd had a busyish day working at Royal Perth Hospital, but in the grand scheme of things, it was a very normal day in healthcare that I'd been experiencing for years. I woke the next day and felt horribly fatigued, lethargic and achy. I'd slept well as usual, but just felt as though I was coming down with a virus (which I wasn't) and wasn't up to getting out of bed. I called in sick to work and spent the rest of the day moving between sleeping in bed to being slumped and drowsy in my lounge chair.

This same routine was to rerun the following day until I finally picked up and resumed the swing of things again two days later. Reassuringly, I never had another incident quite that bad again, but having to rest was boring and a bit depressing, particularly on those days when the sun was shining and it was beautiful outside. I remember having "Sliding Doors" like moments in my mind, imagining what my altered reality might have been like had I not been diagnosed. My parallel reality sometimes felt mindblowing.

Although, I eventually found a rhythm where I could better pace myself and my activities. If I worked one day, I'd leave exercise for the next non-working day. If I was heading out for dinner with friends, I would sleep or rest for a couple of hours prior to going to make sure I was alert and clear-minded enough to be able to have fun and engage with others. Of course, these strategies made me look normal on the outside like the rest of the gang, but the preparation took more effort than people would have realised. My energy levels did improve by three or so years after treatment (this may have been delayed due to another three or so surgeries, and more noticeable given my active lifestyle). Although easier said than done, the key was clearly to remain patient.

Another longer-term issue that I'd need to contend with was an alteration in my heart function. It seemed that my heart muscle strength had reduced after chemotherapy and radiation therapy (undertaken prior to the deep inspiratory breath hold technique that is now available), and I could not exercise to the same high intensity and high level of fitness that I had prior to treatment. Having only had a cardiac stress test and no pre-treatment exercise test, the change that I was experiencing was unable to be quantified, but needless to say it was significant for me and my active lifestyle.

Now when I exercised, I'd get to a point of exertion that I couldn't get over—it was like a ceiling effect that I could no longer push beyond. Friends who I had been on par with now zipped past me when swimming, cycling, and trekking in the hills and although I was giving it my all, I now felt restrained. My lungs had more to give as did my muscles, but my heart could no longer match them. It was hard to get my head around the changes, but when I came to feel bad about it, I'd then feel spoiled, given that I had been lucky to still be alive. My cardiologist reassured me that exercise would be good for me, and that I had no limitations on what I was allowed to do, but it was a change that I would have preferred not to have, especially given my career and hobbies being built around my passion for exercise.

I stayed committed to my rehabilitation and within time, entered a 4km open water swim which was a great achievement. I came in towards the back of the pack compared to the top third where I'd been prior to treatment. But considering I'd swum without my latissimus dorsi and other compromised chest muscles, on top of the chemo and radiation treatment I'd had, it was a good effort. Exercising would remain a mental challenge often, however, I realised along the way, that I'd now have to accept the difference, and try to find a way to simply miss my old self on this one.

There were upsides of this more difficult time though, and one of them was definitely my dog Ebony. When I rested up in bed, she would regularly come into my bedroom every half hour or so, prop herself on my bed with her front paws and check that I was ok. It really was gorgeous having her by my side bringing her energy, positivity and affection. The other big positives were having the opportunity to spend fun times with family and friends. They were definitely the wind beneath my wings, keeping an eye on me, and reminding me what I was about especially when things got shakey.

Conclusion

So, although it looked like my cancer journey was all over once the visible changes like baldness and looking pale were gone, there were still quite a few treatment changes to have to confront. I'd had happy, joyful and fun times spaced over these first few years, but though I'd started looking good on the surface, my disempowerment and struggles would remain under the radar in ways that others didn't notice or couldn't understand. I was now living in a body that needed more TLC and rehabilitation than I would have first thought. It was a world understood to be of challenge in the cancer space, yet a little known one to others in the outside world. The key was to try to keep the faith, keep living life as much as possible, keep exercising and sleeping well, keep the courage and keep the inner light shining, even when it felt dark.

"Keep your eyes on the sun, and you will not see the shadows"
—Australian Aboriginal Proverb.

5.

The Youth Interface. Realities And Challenges.

"Vulnerability is not winning or losing; it's having the courage to show up and be seen when we have no control over the outcome."
—Dr. Brené Brown.

The Realities and Challenges of Youth

Thankfully, breast cancer diagnoses are not common in younger women. Only around 2%, or 1 in 50 of all breast cancers, are diagnosed in women under 35 in Australia. Young women with breast changes have also had issues being taken seriously with some medical practitioners. They have sometimes found themselves being sent away and told it's all ok. Statements quite commonly expressed have included, *"it's just your hormones," "it's probably just a benign lump like a fibroadenoma,"* and *"don't worry as your cancer history is on your father's side of the family."* Even today, some practitioners remain unaware that paternal family cancer histories are just as important as maternal when it comes to breast and ovarian cancer history. Consequently, even when young women have done the right thing by presenting early, their diagnoses have still occurred later than is ideal, having detrimental effects on their outcomes.

Women under 40 currently need to find their breast cancer either by self-detection or through examinations performed by medical practitioners, unless they are under the care of high risk cancer clinics. The result sadly, is that many young women will therefore continue to be diagnosed at a later stage with more advanced disease. They will also often be diagnosed with more aggressive tumours, so survival rates are lower than those of our older breast cancer counterparts. In the 20 to 39-year age bracket, breast cancer incidence and death rates remain the highest compared to other cancers in this same age bracket (Fidler et al., 2017). Breast cancer is also one of the most common cancers diagnosed during pregnancy (Ndlela et al., 2018). Thus, diagnoses at this life stage remain very problematic and more complex.

Being diagnosed in any stage of life has its challenges, but to say that one will know what it's like for a 31-year-old because you know someone who was diagnosed in her 70s for example, is more than likely going to miss the mark. I have been aware of the hardships faced by women at many life stages, including those of my grandmother, but despite the horrid cruelty of a cancer diagnosis in any life stage, the stark contrast and challenge that myself and my contemporaries experienced should not be underestimated.

Although context isn't black and white between age brackets, younger women generally find themselves being less supported physically, emotionally and financially. The support network is invariably less available, with our friends finding sustaining support difficult when they are already working full-time and/ or managing hectic young families around the clock. For many of our friends also, it can be their first up close and personal cancer experience, given that cancer is typically a disease associated with aging. Many young women may also be single, or in newly formed partnerships or marriages and thus less resilient to the swings and punches that cancer can bring. Young women may also have been diagnosed when pregnant, breastfeeding, or with young children. So, breast cancer has so many unique direct and secondary effects for young women, particularly when considering the many social, physical and emotional factors and perspectives.

For me, living alone and being single made my experience different. My friends and family were wonderful, taking the great initiative to call, dropping in to check up on me, inviting me to catch-ups, and so forth. They were also very generous ears on the end of the phone, bringing in the much-needed humour and welcomed distraction. But only a limited number were privy to the smaller, but nevertheless, significant things that I was going through that would have otherwise been seen if not living alone. There were so many sequelae of events after cancer treatment not worth articulating to others, so when they are seen by someone co-habitating with us day to day, this person gains more insight into the real deal and has more opportunity to help here and there, using their initiative and instincts. Although being in relationships during treatment will have it's own set of challenges and hurdles along the way (especially if in an unideal one), if in a stable and supportive relationship, it is probably easy to underestimate what a huge help it can be when facing cancer. For those of us who walk this path as single people, it can be all to clear.

The Financial Realities

As it does for many young people, my diagnosis came when I was fragile and exposed financially, and not yet at a more established and resilient financial platform to face my treatment pathway. I was without many assets or security behind me and of course, was the sole breadwinner. My income was also humble, especially from having to work part-time during and after treatment. So, by in large, I could often hardly rub more than a few dollars together beyond paying my mortgage and other core essential bills for at least the first few years after diagnosis. The bills kept coming too, even increasing with the addition of the medical ones. It certainly wasn't a comfortable situation to be in.

Managing cashflow was like trying to get jigsaw pieces to fit together. Before my diagnosis, I looked into income protection insurance but had unfortunately felt that it was an expense that I just couldn't justify, so there was no assistance from that avenue. I'd exhausted my sick leave after my first surgery, so I would have to be on my own two feet from that point on. I had considered selling my home and moving to a unit after chemotherapy ceased, but calculated that the sale would have probably put me more behind after paying all of the expenses. My next port of call was my superannuation, but that would not have gone very far either.

So although I ended up making ends meet, it was a constant job to try to get my work and finance life to fit together, especially around surgeries, and although I worked so hard to keep things afloat, I would eventually need to ask for help from my family a couple of times in those first few years. They were always willing to lend a hand, but the regular cashflow week by week would always remain an issue. Getting my finances back on track would prove to take a number of years and a lot of stamina.

Re-entering the Relationships Scene

Re-entering the intimate relationship scene after diagnosis and treatment was also an interesting experience. The dating game was now a new territory to confront and found me trying to pick up from where I had left off back in 2006. I now felt like a liability deep down, contributing to a loss of confidence and a feeling of fragmentation under my own skin. I had come to feel less worthy of things after cancer. But, it was up to me to face my fears and change the way I perceived things. No none else could do the work for me. So, about one and a half to two years after my diagnosis, I knew the time had come to get back onto the horse and regain that lost confidence and disempowerment, by getting out there instead of just thinking about it. I had quickly worked out on the dating scene too, that people would generally be pretty ok with my cancer situation when I was, particularly the kind of person that I was searching for. So although I knew that I now had my negatives, I was the only one who could remind others in the world of my positives.

Not long after initial treatment ceased, some friends and acquaintances asked me if I'd met anyone nice, *"yet."* I appreciate that people may have simply been trying to make conversation and that it was just something to say and break the ice, but it made me realise how limited people's understanding could be and the smorgasbord of impacts that we needed to confront. I used to joke with my friends saying that if I met someone really nice and he suggested catching up again, I'd say, *"That sounds great, yes I'd love to catch up, but look, I need to have my ovaries removed next week...and having said that, I had my breasts removed a few years ago as well. Just so we're both on the same page!"* We'd have a good laugh at how ridiculous it all sounded, but such was the reality. It was an insane context. When meeting new people, I'd also have to think about when I'd drop the cancer bomb into our conversations, often feeling that I would be deceiving them until I finally let it all out and put my cards on the table. There was a bit to have to carry when getting back out there.

In my search to meet my partner in and out of crime, I certainly dated a few frogs in those earlier years, that's for sure. My first experience of dating was with a guy who was also a physio but had recently moved into the business world. He seemed quite nice, so after meeting up, we were looking to schedule another time to catch up. I still had short scissor cut hair, which of course, was a bit out on a limb compared to the usual style for a woman in her 30s at that time. During a phone conversation, he said out of the blue, *"To be honest, the idea of sitting across the dinner table from a woman who has hair shorter than mine isn't particularly attractive."* I was stunned by his brazenness. Sure, he hadn't yet known that I'd had chemotherapy the year before as of yet, but his attention to my superficial physical look so early on in the piece gave me a good warning to get the hell out of there. So, I did! When you're pushed out of the world of the majority like you can be with cancer, you can certainly see with more clarity the good in people and the bad in people!

I also met another man not long after my first reconstruction surgery through a friend. To my surprise and the surprise of my friend, this man seemed to want to take things very quickly. His moves would soon have me feeling vulnerable and unsafe, so I knew that he wasn't for me. But I also realised how I had a way to go to feel ok as a woman again under my own skin and would need to do more work to get there. Time would prove that getting back into a relationship would take some time, and I wasn't ready to meet my Mr. Right for a while longer yet. But I had good times getting out and did have a chance to meet some really good people. These two just weren't going to be him.

The Childbearing and Young Cosmesis Interface

As a young woman who'd had breast cancer, I'd find myself frequently in the milieu of the childbearing, parenting and breastfeeding interface after my diagnosis. It was always a confronting space given that I'd needed to forfeit the gift of breastfeeding and was hanging in by a thread in relation to being able to childbear or indeed parent. I recall one confronting occasion, not long after my mastectomies and part one of my reconstruction surgery. A friend had come over to visit with her newborn baby. We had been having a good chat when she realised that her baby needed feeding. Breastfeeding was something that I had given up after having my mastectomies for BRCA1 management, but as the loss was invisible, few would have necessarily thought to spare a thought. With no ill intent, of course, she started to breastfeed.

I wasn't ready to see and confront my loss so soon after my surgery and felt nauseous and, to some degree, traumatised seeing the situation unfold in front of me. Being gracious and probably a bit confused, I stayed in the room and continued to talk to her as though nothing had happened, but the experience sent my head into a bad spin for some time. I admit it was an awkward situation, and there were hardly guidebooks around to help one navigate these sorts of situations. Though in hindsight, I wish at the very least I'd taken some control pragmatically, and had relocated into another room. I worked out as time moved on that all I needed to feel ok, was for each of us to cloak these difficult situations with consideration and a sense of compassion, either in word or in gesture. It said *"I know what you must be going through and how you might be feeling,"* and consequently would help take away the awkwardness, prevent me from mentally tripping up, and help me to keep moving.

People would also often think that my surgery was one and the same as having breast augmentation. I understood why, when the women having this surgery were typically my vintage. But, the breast augment procedure was so different from that of breast reconstruction, technically, physically, psychologically and otherwise. One added to a breast to enhance its size and shape with augments, whereas reconstruction came after the trauma of cancer, and the need to build up an entire breast from ground zero after mastectomy. Not all reconstructions would necessarily turn out looking as pretty as a cosmetic one might either, given that after breast cancer surgery, the skin overlying the breast was often tighter or scarred from prior surgery, lymph node removal and/ or radiation. So I was not a fan of hearing my surgery described as cosmetic, however I would have to contend with the breast cosmesis interface quite a lot over the years from my diagnosis.

Post-operatively in mid-2009, following my part two exchange surgery for my reconstruction, the interface of cosmesis and reconstruction would be lived out once again in real-time. I had been somewhat pushed to the limit at that stage in the timeline, and had been keen to minimise situations that might set me off emotionally or mentally. I had been allocated a two-person room and ended up sharing with a young lady around my age who'd just had breast augment surgery. As I lay in bed contemplating the intensity of my last couple of years, it was party time for her. She spent the morning ringing numerous friends, talking to them about how great her breasts looked, and having a constant stream of friends come to visit. The horrible thing was that I couldn't escape from hearing it, being connected to all sorts of monitoring equipment, drains and infusions. So, Mum and

I asked the nurses if I could kindly move rooms. Thankfully, although the party time celebrations continued, the nursing staff moved her, so it was finally quiet, and I could focus on my recovery and be at peace again.

When I reflect now about my experience, it made me realise how it's easy for organisations to underestimate the impact of health conditions on our psychological and emotional health, and therefore overlook putting processes in place to ensure maximal recovery and wellbeing of their patients. To me, my co-sharing arrangement after this particular surgery, should have been avoided. It exemplified my loss at a time when I wasn't going to be ready for it, when ideally, it should have been helping to cushion the blow.

In 2009, I had also started managing my ovarian cancer risk given that the breast side of things were now mostly sorted except for a few benign issues. After my mastectomies, I was put on the oral contraceptive pill to try to stabilise my wobbly post treatment hormones, as well as to reduce my ovarian cancer risk (the latter is now not recommended). I was also referred for an ovarian ultrasound (now not recommended) and a CA-125 ovarian cancer biomarker blood test (now not recommended as a screening test for women with no symptoms (Cancer Council Australia, 2020)).

In the year or so following my BRCA1 diagnosis, I remember calling the gynae ultrasound clinic to make an appointment. A lovely lady answered and, when looking at her schedule, asked, *"When are you due?"* *"...I'm not,"* I responded. I was a bit startled. When I arrived at the clinic, I again felt like a fish out of water, tripping on some children's toys as I entered the clinic and sitting between three or four pregnant women around my age, them on their way to successful motherhood, and me with a liability or risk of cancer and probable infertility. Again, I was in "no man's land" with few knowing my deal. My saviours would again be the health professionals who mentored and supported me, and for that, I was forever grateful. But, this was the gig of having cancer so young. We would generally need to just get used to it, and try to get on with things as much as I could.

Conclusion

The timing of this disease and the complications that follow aren't kind for young women. Just as we wanted and needed our breasts and ovaries, many of us would have to confront the decision to have them removed. Remaining forward thinking propelled me on, as did trying to let unhelpful thoughts and emotions come and move on. The key was to avoid getting bogged down in the adversity, particularly as the adversities increased in number. So I tried to consciously focus on creating and finding the life that I desperately aspired to live. And that would take tenacious resolve and ongoing commitment, but those before me had shown me that it could be done.

6.
Another Family Cancer Diagnosis. Ongoing Surgeries.

———————•———————•———————

"Don't give up. Don't lose hope."
—Christopher Reeve.

Not long after our own diagnoses with cancer and our surgeries to reduce our cancer risks, mutation carriers will often need to confront other family members being diagnosed and be around to help during their cancer treatments as well. For me, 2012 would again be a tough old ride seeing my cousin's breast cancer diagnosis. But, Christopher Reeve was right. There was never any time to give up, nor lose hope. We'd have to keep our eyes on the sun and not see the shadows. This was just the way that the BRCA1 cookie crumbled.

My Cousin, Gem

My cousin Gem had been about five when her Mum, Merrel, had breast cancer. I can only imagine that the impact that Merrel's breast cancer had on her was profound. Although Merrel survived, closely experiencing her Mum's illness as she undertook arduous treatments and navigated her ongoing recovery into the medium and longer term, would have been a challenge to anyone at the best of times. At the time of Merrel's diagnosis, there was little help, with no real support services or counselling that we now see. For those affected, and their families and loved ones, they were mostly left to their own devices to "just get on with it", process the losses, accept the changes and cope with the aftermath. In Merrel and Gem's case also, the support within the family was light on, due to Gem's father moving out not long after her birth, on top of the loss of our Grandma only eight years prior to Merrel's diagnosis.

Gem felt her breast lump, also at 31. Her life had however, seen some twists and turns, and she had unfortunately come to have some issues with drugs that she was trying desperately hard to kick. When I turned up at her first surgical appointment as a support person after not having seen her for some years, I soon realised that I had stepped back in time to 1984, all those decades before. It was like déjà vu—the past was back even though so much had happened since then. History was repeating itself, and again we were hearing the words, "You have breast cancer."

I supported Gem through her breast cancer treatment pathway, as with her father long gone and her brother Tony based overseas, there wasn't as much family help on deck to see her through. Given that I knew the breast cancer scene having been there and done that in the recent past, I was glad that I could help. But I felt incredibly raw and deeply sad attending appointments. It was also a lot to bear walking alongside Gem in it's own right, let alone on top of juggling a few of my own issues that had cropped up in my own backyard. There were a few stumbles for Gem, but within time she made it through her surgery, which was a huge relief to us all.

After Gem's surgery, we went "breast prosthesis shopping" together, which although horrible to have to do, it ended up being fun in some sort of way too. It was also good to touch base outside of the hospital walls and the cancer consultations, which were always intense. Unfortunately following our prosthesis visit, Gem then found out that chemotherapy was off the cards as the delay between her diagnosis and presenting for treatment had been too long, so the benefit was seen to be too small to be worthwhile. It was now up to Gem's body to fend for itself. I can't imagine the anguish and inner struggles that both Merrel and Gem had to confront during this time.

For me, when I reflect back about Gem's diagnosis, I found that I had to give as much as we could to help, not only for her, but also for me too. We'd lived through Merrel's diagnosis together, me as a nine year old and Gem as a five year old, and again it felt like it was us versus this bastard disease. It seemed that it was also just going to be the two of us this time round. We were in it together and had to be in it together. Such is the connection of genetic diseases. It's not just about us alone, but it's about us together.

Ongoing Breast Surgeries

Around the time of Gem's diagnosis, I also had some further breast surgeries. Not long before her diagnosis, I had developed some breast lumps that radiology, unfortunately, didn't like the look of. They ended up both being benign, one being a fatty lump called a lipoma and the other being a neuroma or a lump of sensitive nerve tissue. These had likely been a result of my previous breast surgeries.

Due to changes in my right nipple as well, I had further surgery a couple of years later. This time, nothing looked suspicious, however, the scans had appeared to have some residual breast tissue left behind, so my surgeon wanted this removed as, *"I was still young"* and my risk for cancer, even with this smaller amount of supposed breast tissue, was still unsatisfactory. On reflection, I suspect that my right nipple had deformed and deviated due to the more intensive yoga and swimming that I had been doing. My latissimus nerve supply had been aberrant hence the muscle was still partially activating on the right breast, so the skin was also pulled and tugged when using my arms, thus likely resulting in the apparent tissue and nipple change. Each surgery that I had would, of course, add a level of stress, particularly on balancing my recovery and work around it, but although not anticipated all those years ago at diagnosis, I haven't been alone. I have since seen many women go through recurrent unexpected breast surgeries for many reasons as well.

Ovarian Surgery

2013 was the year that I was referred to see my gynae oncologist. It was the year following Gem's diagnosis and six years since my initial breast cancer diagnosis. My risk of developing ovarian cancer had started to rise significantly, and my poor ovaries had started to show signs of ovarian decline, medically known as "premature ovarian failure." I had wanted to hang onto them for as long as possible for hormonal and fertility purposes, so I had held my nerve for those six years and had made it to 37.

By this stage, having already had about six breast surgeries, I considered myself a veteran of the surgical knife, and thought I knew what it was now all about. I therefore thought that the salpingo-oophorectomy surgery (removal of the fallopian tubes and ovaries) would be a relative walk in the park, but time would prove how wrong I would be. Stuart, my surgeon, was very understanding, empathetic, reassuring and kind. One of his specific areas of special interest was managing high-risk women such as myself, so it was very palpable that he had much insight into the challenges that mutation carriers like myself faced. He had an excellent calming bedside manner, and I had a high level of confidence in him and his team's care.

However, despite this, I found myself feeling more vulnerable than I had with my breast surgeries. For me, my ovaries represented the nucleus of my womanhood. They were more central and core to my sense of femininity than my breasts had been, so confronting the losses that would come from this surgery made me realise that I had more to lose this time around than I had before. Ironically, the laparoscopic, or keyhole surgery, was known for being minimally invasive, but for me emotionally, it felt maximally invasive. Although, unlike the breast surgery, there was no visible loss on the outside, it however, would prove to be an insult of forfeited promise on the inside.

After the surgery, my sister Sil and Alice (now aged six) came to visit me. I had been dosed up on the strong painkiller methadone, which had knocked me out quite strongly and made me unable to stop my eyes from rolling. I am sure that I looked a bit different and scary. Not expecting to see me look washed-out, poor Alice had a look of fear when she first saw me. She was motionless and stood staring at me. On seeing this, my sister Sil promptly jumped in, explaining, *"You know when you're waking up in the morning and how you feel a bit tired and sleepy? Aunty Trinie is just feeling a bit like that."* One really horrible reality of cancer is that we can't always protect each other, let alone our young folk, from the ugliness of it all the time. We can only do our best by listening and keeping an eye on it. Thankfully, Alice was fine with Sil's explanation, but the experience did make me realize what having a diagnosis in this age bracket could really be like.

Though the surgery itself went well despite the post-op methadone hiccup, within a couple of weeks, it was evident that the balance of my body had certainly been given a smashing. It can be easy to underestimate how much influence our female hormones have on so many tissues and organs of the body until we no longer have them. I was put on a low dose of hormone replacement using an Estradot patch post-operatively, however it soon became clear that this was insufficient. I had trouble sleeping, and my cognitive and word-finding ability was impaired. I felt like I was "a sandwich short of a picnic." These changes made me feel very exposed, particularly in the workplace, including in the university setting. My emotions had also simultaneously dropped to be very low, as though I'd jumped off a cliff from relative happiness to some sort of muddied despair or confusion. I wasn't feeling too much joy for the world. Given these intolerable changes, Stuart increased the hormone replacement patch dose. Although my sleep, cognition, and emotions were back beautifully, the HRT then induced an outbreak of horrid cystic acne over my entire back. It was proving to be a fine balancing act to get my hormone levels right!

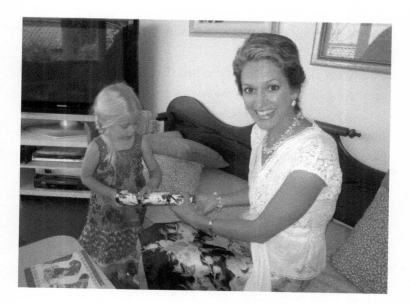

Alice and I

I also had a Mirena IUD inserted to supply local progesterone for uterine health in the hope of keeping everything ticking, just in case my hopes to be able to have children were to materialise.

However, within a couple of years from my gynae surgery, the hormone replacements and the unstable hormonal levels that I was trying to get right, ended up causing a uterine polyp. Again, I required another surgery (number eight or so) to investigate the issue further and remove it. This stopped the bleeding of course, but I then realised that my hormone replacement would now be insufficient to "hold the fort" and keep my endometrial lining under control. So, I would now have to have pseudo-periods every month or two (given that I had no ovaries) to keep things under control. This reality made me realize why Gynaecologists usually recommend that the uterus be removed at the time of oophorectomies. The trio really did come as a package and the uterus really did need the ovaries to tell it what to do.

Eventually through trial and error, thanks to both Stuart and my menopausal specialist, my hormone replacement came to be as close to good as it was going to be, so even though it was still imperfect, it was functional and had me feeling good, sleeping well and acne-free. There were other changes, particularly with my skin drying out and my hair thinning, but thankfully, my bone density managed to stay on track, which is the most important thing, especially given my ongoing hope for survival for the decades ahead.

After the gynae surgery, I then had to manage some issues from a sexual health perspective due to hormonal loss and hence, sexual functioning decline. With help from sexual health experts, I came to manage things ok, even though I much preferred my pre-menopausal self. I realized too that sexual changes would prove to add another consideration and potential hurdle when entering any new relationships going forward, but I needed to keep the faith and keep my empowerment, turning my liability into an asset if you will. I had taken my fate into my own hands by having the surgery in the first place, and most importantly, I would still claim my turf as a gorgeous woman in my head and heart, even if I was now a bit different in my body.

Conclusion

The milieu of ongoing cancers with BRCA1 could certainly reduce the social fabric within any family, having to cope with ongoing intergenerational losses and traumas that come with the disease, whilst also having to confront our own personal challenges from our own diagnoses. For me personally survival continued to be a privilege, and although I didn't always take to the fallout of BRCA1 kindly, I also knew that my grandmother's life would have been spared if she'd had this genetic and medical technology around during her lifetime. Now having had my oopherectomies, I was now looking hopeful that the bulk of the BRCA1 fallout would finally lie behind me. It had been quite a journey to survive, recover and to try to keep my dreams alive.

7.

The Journey Of Infertility. The Ultimate Invisible Loss.

●—————————————●

"We must accept finite disappointment, but never lose infinite hope."
—Dr. Martin Luther King, Jr

Despite the positive effect that the chemotherapy treatment had on my survival, it came with a substantial negative one. The decade following my diagnosis would see my infertility being brought down by degrees, with my hope shifting from having my own child to pursuing donated eggs from my cousin to being offered embryos from friends. Living with infertility suspended for over a decade within the era of fertility was an indescribably hard interface to have to live within. For those of us who had cancer, our infertility would not be a loss in isolation either, coming on top of a number of other losses that had already come our way. But, I could not lose infinite hope, and the gift of being asked to be my nephew Lachie's godmother in 2009 was certainly a wonderful and touching kindness.

Chemotherapy and Infertility

Prior to treatment, I was informed that my fertility would be reduced due to chemotherapy's irreparable effects on the ovaries. The reason was that at birth, we are born with a finite number of egg cells. The chemotherapy damaged these fastly dividing cells, hence the number of available eggs had reduced significantly, leaving young women like myself closer to infertile or fully infertile after treatment. At the time of my diagnosis in 2007, I wasn't referred to see a fertility specialist, presumably because at this point in time, the IVF process remained very tenuous with only a 2% success rate of having a live birth (Sample, 2007). According to the Human Fertilisation and Embryo Authority in the UK, the success rate across the board now sits at around 21% (Gurtin, 2019). So a consultation with a fertility specialist is very much encouraged for most younger women if diagnosed at the current time.

In the hope of preserving my fertility, I was prescribed Zoladex (Goserelin) injections during my chemotherapy. These were given monthly into my abdomen to shut down my ovaries further, taking me into even deeper menopause than the chemotherapy did alone. At the time, this course of treatment held promise regarding fertility preservation in theory, but it was still largely experimental. Research published eight years later would demonstrate positive improvements in fertility (Moore et al., 2015), so in theory, the Zoladex treatment that I had should have made at least some difference to my fertility level. However in 2016, it was found that healthy BRCA1 mutation carriers have a 25% lower fertility rate at 35 than women without the mutation of the same age (Phillips et al., 2016), so it may well have been that the tide had already been against me, even without the superimposed chemotherapy treatment.

BRCA1 Issues with Fertility

The other concern over my head since finding out that I was a mutation carrier was the potential risk of passing on the BRCA1 gene mutation to my child. The risk of inheritance was 50% as the mutation carried an autosomal dominant pattern of inheritance. In my mind, the risk of passing on the mutation was horrid. However, the only other options posed to me had their imperfections ethically, practically, and with matters of the heart. The thought of potentially letting conception take its course with its associated risks wasn't a great prospect. Our loss as a family due to BRCA1 had been too great and had gone on for too long, but the idea of undertaking a fairly new technology called Pre-Implantation Genetic Diagnosis (PGD) had its maze of challenges too.

For the first few years after diagnosis, the notion of having children seemed a long way away. Many of my resources were limited and Mr. Right hadn't turned up as of yet, but I still wanted to make sure that I left no stone unturned as fertility was important to me, as having a family had always been something that I had wanted to experience and do in my life. So, to be a step ahead of the game in 2008, I looked further into the option of undertaking PGD. PGD was an IVF procedure that involved identifying unaffected embryos free of the BRCA1 mutation and preferentially using them instead of affected ones at the time of implantation. To use this technology back in 2008, I would have needed to submit an application for approval to the Reproductive Technology Council of Western Australia (WA). A test would have been needed to be developed, which alone could have taken up to 12 months, and if it was not possible to undertake in WA, I would have needed to travel interstate. So, although the PGD option was appealing, it looked like it would be yet another big hurdle to get over if I was able to do it and if I was to choose it.

Decisions such as undertaking PGD are certainly very personal for anyone who happens to find themselves in this situation. From where I stood, I tended more towards a stance of prevention being better than a cure. PGD offered the opportunity for BRCA1 mutation carriers with that step alone to prevent the ongoing intergenerational trauma, loss and adversity that our families invariably experience generation after generation. As it would turn out, the option of using PGD would be a decision-making concept that would not go any further, but nevertheless, one that was worth exploring.

Ovarian Decline and The Search for Donor Eggs

Before my oophorectomy surgery, I noticed that things had been starting to change hormonally, so I went and had my fertility biomarker levels (Anti-Mullerian Hormone or AMH) as well as my oestrogen, progesterone and testosterone levels tested. I was peri-menopausal, and my AMH levels were unquantifiable as they were below 1, when normal values were between 15 to 30. So, essentially my ovaries were well into their 50s biologically, even though chronologically they were only 36. This meant that there would definitely be no chance of having my own child. With this low production of oestrogen and progesterone hormones from my ovaries, I would also run the increased risk of difficulty sustaining a pregnancy.

After my gynae surgery where my uterus was spared, the next option along the pathway for having children was to source donor eggs. My older sister was out because of a health issue that had cropped up, so I approached a cousin who very generously stepped up to the plate. She was 34, looked a bit like me but was taller and more tanned than me, so I thought this might not be so bad! My cousin had some provisional testing done, and unfortunately, she too had a low AMH coming in at around 4. So that option ended with her also being infertile. I was devastated for her, especially as it had been through my actions that she had come to know about this result, but she seemed to take the findings in stride and accepted that it was just how it was.

A few years later, I was offered another dash of hope when a lovely friend and her husband approached me. They offered me some of their IVF embryos after successfully completing their family with their two gorgeous kids. I was overjoyed by their generosity and gratefully accepted their incredibly kind offer. To bring this opportunity to life from a practical point of view, however, I knew there would be many other considerations that would need addressing too. If or when the time arose, I would need to have a conversation with a new partner about having children that wouldn't be biologically ours. The child's parents would also be new acquaintances for my future partner, so he would have to be comfortable with both them and the arrangement. But still, it gave me a glimmer of hope (about a 5% probability of success), in a space that had prior to that, felt hopeless.

Social Consequences of Infertility

Often, when out and about, it was also natural that I would be asked if I had children. It was a simple conversation starter for some and general curiosity and interest for others. I found that with not having kids, it was usually assumed that I just hadn't wanted them or that I'd left it "too late," so I would usually respond by saying, *"Not yet, unfortunately."* Then by in large, the conversation wouldn't go any further.

But, from time to time I have also unfortunately come across people who have viewed parenthood like a club that one either belonged to or they didn't. As motherhood clearly isn't a human right afforded to all, coming across these situations could be frustrating. I developed a couple of ways to try to handle these times as I came across them. I would either decide to just let the situation go, or if I felt like there was a window of opportunity to educate others about the challenges of cancer and infertility, I would gently but honestly place my cards on the table. Although the latter wasn't always easy to do, I felt that it might help others to understand the realities that we found ourselves in and I also hoped that ultimately, it might make the road easier for the next person.

When I look back, my 30s and 40s haven't been particularly easy. It is a time when those of us challenged by fertility are surrounded by many people being pregnant, showing their baby photos, having baby showers, christenings and so on. The interface of the consumerist machines of the Mother's and Daughter's Day movements can also be a challenge when confronting infertility in this childbearing age-bracket. I hope in time that we see a shift in this space as well as a broader acknowledgement of the diversity out there, and a movement towards more inclusivity. In view of this, I decided a few years back to have my own symbolic mother's days as a mother of my furry baby, and as a carer and mentor for my patients. There is no reason why the definition of motherhood can't be broadened.

I've also tried and I hope succeeded, to keep my courage when around others who have become pregnant, new parents or grandparents. I've tried to place myself in other people's shoes, and join them in their excitement and joy, rather than revealing my invisible loss, or allowing myself the indulgence of becoming overly self-focused with it all. Sometimes though, I would need to keep to myself and do the "hermit technique," as I just didn't always have the strength to face things. I'd also try other tactics, such as making myself busy with my work and projects, and distracting myself by focusing on other things in my life. These strategies, however, would only get me to a certain point. At the end of the day, some level of acceptance of my infertility would prove to be the only true remedy. And this has thankfully been easier to do with the grace of time.

Adoption and Fostering

When people have discovered that I was infertile, a common follow up question is to ask whether I thought about adopting or fostering children. Adoption in Australia is almost impossible, and comes with a huge expense, stress, uncertainty and much hard work. Waiting for several years is not uncommon either and children will often possess cultural and ethnic differences and may also have special needs (Intercountry Adoption Australia, 2020). After a cancer diagnosis, agencies also need to discuss possible adoption with your doctors. They may need to perform a medical examination to determine the risk of the cancer returning or for mutation carriers, another cancer developing, as well as your ability to raise a child (Cancer Council NSW, 2020). So there are many hoops to have to jump through, making it an even more difficult option than it already is, for anyone who has had cancer. The context of cancer and fostering is not one that would necessarily be easy, even at the best of times. So with the context of my diagnosis and the impacts that it has had, unfortunately adopting or fostering children has not been something that I have felt adequately equipped or positioned to do.

Conclusion

The consequences of infertility are irreversible, profound and last a lifetime. Living with infertility isn't a straightforward or comfortable milieu by any means, particularly in the childbearing years. But we also need to recognise that it can be a difficult space for all. Ultimately, we need to be able to find a way to navigate the bumps on the road of this complex path, and as we do so, maintain the utmost compassion and empathy for each other.

It will help if the broader communications around infertility are shaken up so that conversations can be more open and honest. It will help if both awareness and education of the consequences of infertility become more prevalent in the public space, so that there is improved understanding of the challenges and the loss of promise. This improved understanding would improve healing and would also help to remove the isolation that we all invariably feel.

8.

Relationships With Others. Connection And Tenacity.

•────────────────•

The Importance of Friends

"Many people will walk in and out of your life, but only true friends will leave footprints in your heart."

—Eleanor Roosevelt.

Relationships with both family and friends have been instrumental in helping me move through my cancer experience. One of the most enriching parts of having had cancer, despite it's negatives, has been forming many wonderful relationships with others along the way and, in doing so, learning so much. But relationships have not always been smooth sailing. During and after cancer, I found they could be difficult, often requiring additional patience, loyalty and care than they would have otherwise needed. Some relationships have grown and become stronger after my diagnosis, but I've also lost some friends along the way. When we walk this path too, many of us will need to find a way to cope, given that some of our family members or friends that we meet won't make it. So, all the more reason for making happy memories and holding onto these good times, so that they can live on in our hearts and minds for the years to come.

At the time I was diagnosed, I had limited opportunities to meet contemporary women who'd also had a breast cancer experience like mine and were living in Perth. It was just a matter of time though, and within about four years, I came across some like-minded friends with whom I could share my experiences. Tania, Alysia, Fi and Tracey were positive, articulate, smart and all-around lovely company. Although we were at different stages of managing the fallout of cancer, I felt like I had finally found "home" when we caught up with each other. We understood each other's experiences first-hand, particularly regarding entering new relationships as single women, navigating the financial blows as breadwinners, as well as navigating the physical changes from treatment in our active lives. I found that it was such a relief not having to explain myself or my circumstances. Our friendships were rather able to be based on the foundations of shared experience. It made me realise that friendships with those who understood were worth their weight in gold.

A downside though, would be that I'd have to come to accept that I would end up losing some friends as I went. My first friends to pass were the two friends who walked with me in my first year of cancer treatment. I lost a very good friend when Cam passed from his myeloma in 2011. Along with Libby, we had had many good times together, and his support and friendship through those vulnerable and uncertain times had been a godsend. What Cam had to say had always resonated with me, and made me think in a way that I hadn't before. I had never wanted our friendship to end, but it was wonderful to have at least had the friendship that we'd had for as long as we did. I know that I've been all the richer for having known him.

Some years after her diagnosis, my friend Jude who I'd met in Melbourne in 2007, also passed. She'd eventually found true love, marrying her lovely man Adam, and they had at least a few wonderful years together. I wasn't around in her last years, but the photos that I saw of that time showed a very brave and courageous young woman who kept living life to the fullest right up to the end. Adam walked with her hand in hand through her last days, providing much love and care right to her last moments. I was glad that she'd had some sort of silver lining to her cloud having met Adam, but was so sad that she had got the short straw with her cancer. Jude had not even come close to reaching her potential given all that she could have been. I can only imagine how those close to her must have felt and must still be feeling all these years later.

I would also lose another very special friend called Joe. I met Joe in 2014. She was a beautiful English lady in her late 40s, who was married with two boys. Joe was a passionate paediatric nurse, surf lifesaver and swimmer. She had initially attended my practice, but we had struck a chord with each other, both finding that we had so many common interests as health professionals as well as a passion for open water swimming. Through Joe's encouragement, I got back into swimming competitively. She helped me face my fears and adjust psychologically to my altered abilities after reconstruction, something that I had avoided doing up until I met her. It was a steep learning curve, but we had a lot of fun in the process, entering a number of competitive open water swims, both as a duo team, as well as solo participants.

Although initially diagnosed with early breast cancer, Joe's cancer progressed and metastasized within a few years after diagnosis. From that point on, she confronted one adversity after another with virtually no reprieve. I felt for her and her family, having to endure such a relentless string of heartbreaking losses. Despite this however, even up to her last days, Joe kept her friends close to her. She pushed on hard, which even included dropping a gift into my work in her last week, when she clearly wasn't very well at all.

The thing was that friends meant a lot to Joe. She had such a big heart and had connected with so many people and had even managed to form a strong community of friends in the six years that she and her family had been in Australia. Joe knew what life was all about—good friendships, savouring experiences, having a go and helping others. I learned so much from her, and feel so lucky to have had the chance to have her in my life. But as with Cam, I had just never wanted it to be over.

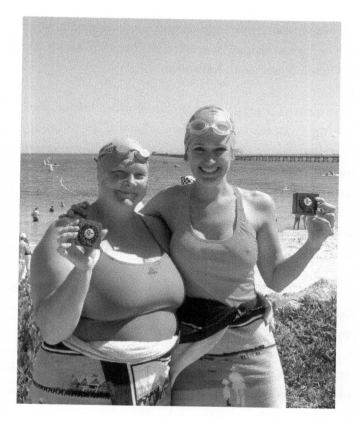

Joe and I

Where there are losses in the cancer space though, we also need to see and invest in the gains. There is something beautiful in the fact that our shared memories live on, and that our friends can stay in our hearts and minds till the end of time. Another gain is being able to continue making memories with friends who have survived their cancers. We sometimes catch up to walk and swim together, and enjoy the double dose of therapy, by enjoying our conversations and chats, as well as enjoying having the chance to exercise and rehabilitate. The support and encouragement we give to each other has helped us reach our potential, and it has also provided an avenue to have fun.

I have also made many good friends from all around the world with my voluntary cancer advocacy work. Even though our individual cancer circumstances and our access to treatments have varied from country to country, we have found a common bond and kinship through our interest in research and our passion to make tomorrow a better day. Together, we have raised the bar to reduce gaps and improve current practices in breast cancer care. It has been a critical step having people who have been there and done that sitting at the decision-making tables, interacting with researchers, health services planners and health care funding organizations, to make sure that we get improvements and progress where it is really needed.

I've found the work really stimulating and productive, and have enjoyed being able to use my unique perspective and experiences to be able to help make tomorrow better for others. It has been particularly empowering seeing more people being able to make decisions regarding their care based on being fully informed about the pros, cons and potential impacts of their decisions, by being able to access more holistic consumer-reviewed information, in contrast to times gone by. It makes me realise how far we've come since consumer advocacy has been integral to the research and health care processes.

Genetic Mutation Relationship Challenges

Genetic diseases can add another level of strain on relationships, particularly within families who carry inherited genetic mutations. The multiple layers of impact and challenge can also sometimes be hard to understand, even for those of us with the gene mutations. When we walk the genetic terrain, I've learned that it's important to remain connected and patient of everyone's individual journeys, by allowing issues and learnings to evolve and resolve in their own way, and their own time.

For me, being the only BRCA1 carrier besides Dad in my immediate family, there were family times when I would acutely feel aware of what BRCA1 and cancer had got in the way of. Of course, my family would help as much as was humanly possible to minimise me feeling this way, but I sometimes felt like a fish out of water and it was hard to put my fish back into it. It was like I was stuck in a holding pattern, away from the prosperity and growth that I would have otherwise invariably been experiencing. I could do little to accelerate the steps I needed to take. Having been diagnosed so young, unless I had been prepared to have my oophorectomies back in 2008 at 32 with the consequent lower success rate of fertility and an even earlier onset of menopause, I needed to shoulder being stuck in limbo, until all going well, I could meet my Mr Right. It was a stalemate really. A diagnosis, even in the latter childbearing years or later 40s, would have more than likely been kinder on this front.

The times I found hardest were during festive family times like Christmases, with some years being more difficult than others. Family times were important, but the backdrop of these times' apparent happiness could be a strain, particularly when I wasn't feeling my best. One Christmas that comes to mind was the one in 2013 on the back of my infertility and oopherectomies. I recall sitting at the table for a Christmas dinner, wishing that I could miraculously and instantly remove myself from the emotionally confronting time that I was having. I didn't want to make a fuss or make anyone feel horrible as no one had done anything wrong, but at the same time, I just wanted a release from the discomfort and sadness that the festivities were heightening.

Things did pick up, but it took time and a significant dose of strength of character, compassion, courage and maturity from all of us.

I would also unfortunately come to witness the complexities of the BRCA1 journey with others. Some years after diagnosis, I met a lovely young woman diagnosed with breast cancer in her 20s due to the BRCA1 mutation. She said that her father's guilt of passing on the gene mutation was very high, eventually culminating in her parents finding themselves unable to offer their support and visit her in hospital after her reconstruction surgery. The genetic landscape of guilt, loss of control and uncertainty had somehow managed to get to a point where it had pulled her family even further apart. It was so heartbreaking to hear. The courage to show up despite the stresses and strains was evidently a hurdle just too high. Thankfully despite having had some challenges with depression and post traumatic stress disorder, this lovely soul redirected her life into happier times, through the love and support of friends, cancer organizations and with the gift of time, her family. I've really admired her courage to do this. I can only imagine that it must have been incredibly difficult.

I also made another friend who had the BRCA1 gene mutation. She had said that in her family (in contrast to ours), there had been many females with BRCA1 who developed cancer, including her mother, numerous aunts, cousins, nieces and so on. My friend said that down the track, even though so many relatives had been affected by breast cancer, many of them had since passed, so she had come to feel very isolated being one of the few survivors in her family. So it made me realise that even in a sea of inherited cancer diagnoses with BRCA1, many of us could ironically still feel somewhat alone and isolated, for more reasons than might meet the eye— death, few diagnoses, geographical distance, social upheaval, fear and denial. The genetic disease landscape could certainly be complex.

BRCA1 needs us to try to find a place where living with it is ok, no matter how it pans out within our life, or our family unit. After all, it isn't going to go away. Our pasts aren't going to be able to change, and our realities may only be influenced up to a certain point. We need to learn to co-exist with it somehow, keeping it in the background and off to the side when possible, but nevertheless able to deal with it's issues, if and when they arise. It is a juggling act, but we need to find a way.

Counselling Support for Better Relationships

About five years after diagnosis, I decided that professional, impartial and objective help from a counsellor would be a good way to go, particularly on the back of my most challenging fallouts— my BRCA1 diagnosis, my fertility issues and Gem's diagnosis. I found Cynthia, an excellent counsellor and mental health social worker. Cynthia really helped me to understand and shelve my personal issues and emotions around my BRCA1 and cancer diagnoses, and their existential threat. She helped me to find a way to acknowledge and accept the hardships that had come my way. She also helped me reconnect and rebuild a stronger relationship with myself in the midst of the cancer storm, when its upheavals and unpredictable destabilising changes made me feel somewhat lost and uncertain.

After my diagnosis also, I'd more frequently find myself in heightened states of emotions that weren't healthy for either myself or others around me. I'd start to view situations and people through a more polarised lens than I had in the past, rather than seeing things as the mixture of good and bad or light and dark that they really are. Cynthia gave me some tools to soften my gaze by helping me see life in more shades of colour, rather than the more dogmatic black and white viewpoints that had started to emerge in my angst and frustrations.

She helped me come to the realisation that life was about so much more—seeing the good in people even if there was bad, keeping connections with others afloat, and remembering to cut both myself and other people slack. We have to give each other space to learn as we go. The more we lose and the more we are challenged year by year, the more we need to learn, and the more we need to get good at letting go. I've found that practice doesn't always make perfect, as it has sometimes been harder to achieve the more I've had to do it, not the other way round.

So it has been about putting one foot in front of the other, and staying in the arena to give it my very best shot.

Conclusion

Although cancer can be an isolating space, the flipside is that it can be an opportunity to make new friends, to strengthen relationships with ourselves and our loved ones, and to enable us to grow and learn. Meaningful relationships with others also help us to get the most out of our lives and enjoy our precious time here. Relationships cannot be undervalued.

Now, more often than not, counselling and psychological support are very accessible being a referral, website and/ or phone call away. Cancer organisations can also help to take the bumps out of the road and can give us the tools to manage adversity and enable deep understanding and healing. We just need to be brave enough to reach out.

"The best thing to hold onto
in life is each other."
—Audrey Hepburn.

MY STORY

My Learnings Of Hope & Healing

9.

Cancer Communications. The Importance Of Help, Mindset And Empathy.

•————————————•

"I've learned that people will forget what you said, people will forget what you did, but people will never forget how you made them feel."

—Maya Angelou.

When someone we know has been having a tough time, it can be really hard to know what to do or not do, or know what to say or not say. We don't usually have intentions to hurt others or cause harm, however, sometimes it just happens. We don't know what we don't yet know, and we can only learn with the wisdom of hindsight. But at the end of the day, we are more likely to have success with our communications if we consider and respect the needs and feelings of others, and also consider the timing and manner in which we communicate. Here are some lessons and tips that I've learned along the way.

Why Me? How Beliefs Can Harm

I think that anyone who is diagnosed with cancer wonders what went wrong. Cancer rocks us to the core about who we are and what we are about, so searching for meaning or looking at alternative explanations can be something that many of us do. I too questioned this before the confirmation of my genetic diagnosis. However, unfortunately after my cancer diagnosis, it went with the territory that I would hear many people's opinions about why I got breast cancer at a time when few do. Many things said were unfounded or myth-based. I found myself being told what I did and didn't do, think, or didn't think, ate and didn't eat. I hadn't eaten organic food, I had consumed dairy, I'd worn an underwired bra. I'd been stressed, I had held resentment, and I hadn't been breathing properly, so I had toxins build up in my blood and so on. It has also been implied quite a few times, that cancer may have been something that I had *"attracted"* into my life or that my cancer had been a form of *"karma."*

Hearing these reasons was exasperating. They were incorrect, toxic, unhelpful and sometimes harmful. I'd felt that some of these comments exploited my vulnerabilites, given that in part, I felt like I must have somehow been to blame for having become unwell. My advice to others is therefore to leave the causes of getting cancer to the person with cancer, their treating health professionals with their sophisticated intimate knowledge of the complex science of cancer, and those close to them. Everyone is in a unique and highly individualised situation, and few are privy to the many facts at hand. Respect those diagnosed, and view being around this person as an opportunity to grow and learn alongside them. Leave the soul searching and fact finding to them.

The Harm of Comparisons and Being Dismissive

When hearing of others' cancer diagnoses, it's wise to avoid comparing one person's situation with others. From the time of my diagnosis, I found that my situation was compared to someone else with breast cancer, or even to others who had a different type of cancer. These comparisons were at the least an unwanted complication and at worst, harmful, especially when heard in my less resilient moments. At times I also unfortunately found that my cancer situation would be dismissed because I had "only had breast cancer." It made me realise that many of us with cancer could easily be misunderstood, especially for those in a similar situation to mine as the younger adult with high-risk familial cancers. For me and for many, coping with the primary issues associated with more advanced and aggressive cancer diagnoses, alongside the secondary ones such as managing ongoing cancer risks, family planning complications, other cancer diagnoses within the family etc., was no mean feat.

So, the message that people need to know is that cancer comes in all shapes and sizes, and that it is likely that you will know very little about a person's cancer and circumstances that might come with it. Comparisons and assumptions are unhelpful, and can be further isolating. A cancer diagnosis removes people from prosperity and privilege, and it's worth remembering that some may have had even less of these to begin with. So it's really important to listen, learn and support. We can do better!

The Need to Listen and Acknowledge

One of the best ways to facilitate recovery after any health crisis comes with simply being heard and when possible, understood. Although many of my family and friends deserve a gold medal for so selflessly offering their ears and time, I did however also find from time to time, that some people couldn't bring themselves to really hear what was being said.

A couple of these experiences that come to mind occurred just before my mastectomies and reconstructions. I wanted to confront my loss and reach out to others, but it seemed that rather than being listened to, a number of people felt more comfortable controlling the conversation and steering it exclusively to the pluses. I'd hear comments like, *"Just think, they (your breasts) will never sag"* or *"They'll always look great, even as you get older,"* and so on. Perhaps some people were disappointed for me or even unsure about what to say, but all I had really wanted, was for it to be ok to have a bit of airtime and ok to be honest, without the need to protect anyone or run from the truth. I wanted some acknowledgement of some small part of my reality first, including the bad and the ugly, before we plunged into the positives.

We need others to spare us some kindness to try to see our point of view, and to understand our circumstances, feelings, challenges, hopes and dreams. This is the only way, if others are to be able get closer to understanding us and gain insight into who we really are.

The Power of Encouragement

Encouragement goes a long way, even if we're tired and it's hard to give. Sometimes going through cancer or being a carer of someone with cancer is no less remarkable an achievement than winning a prestigious award. The hard work, commitment and perseverance to just get by and move towards tomorrow both during and after cancer can be of the same, if not greater in magnitude. I found that when others gave me words of encouragement, it boosted my ability to cope and boosted my self-worth. Encouragement for many of us lets us know that we are supported, and that our efforts to get through are being noticed. Hearing more encouragement like, *"You're doing well"* and *"You should be proud of yourself getting through all of this,"* etc., would have been such a bonus. Receiving encouragement is very much part of the healing process, more than we might think.

What to Do or Say When You're Lost for Words?

Not long after I finished treatment, I provided some rehabilitation for a lovely young gentleman who had a brain tumour. He unfortunately passed away not long afterwards. I had a frank conversation with his wife who was also an acquaintance of mine. I told her about my being a bit lost for words seeing the losses that so many people had to endure. Nothing that entered my mind seemed quite right to say. She said that what often spoke loudest for her, was other's simply being present. She gained much strength by simply being around others who offered their thoughts and support. She also said, *"You know, it's ok to say, I don't know what to say."* Beyond being genuine, I realised that this simple response also took away the pressure that we can all feel when we awkwardly try and find something fitting to say. It was a pearl of wisdom that I've held onto since.

Doing So Little but at the Right Time, Goes So Far

After meeting so many people who are often at their worst and most fragile state, I have been so surprised at how often we can be helped back on our feet by people around us doing small, kind and considerate things.

I remember in my hardest and loneliest of times that people would have a smile on their face when I walked past them on the street, or would start up a friendly conversation with me when I was walking Ebi. The number of times that these positive exchanges happened just when I needed it was uncanny. Perhaps given I was living alone, these seemingly small but positive connections with aquaintances or strangers would help me more than they might others. But time and time again, they would help me to reset my thinking, sending me down a more positive track mentally and in doing so, lift my spirits. The community really can help in ways that they don't realise, just by going about their daily business and sparing a thought.

Compassion Fatigue

Another challenge that can rear its head, like any disease that has a longer trajectory, is that "compassion fatigue" can slip into play after a longer period of time very easily. This is understandable, no matter how brilliant people are around you. After the intensive treatment for early breast cancer, it's easy for people to want to think that we are "better now" and that life can "go back to normal" because we often start to look good again with more colour in our faces and our hair growing back. However, the many medium-term and longer-lasting side effects aren't yet over, so the situation asks a lot of both ourselves and of those close to us. The reality is, even though others around us may become "fatigued" for us as the "CEOs" of our illness, we can't be afforded the luxury of compassion fatigue. We've just gotta keep going, and going, with the utmost resilience and tenacity. As we do this, we need to remain compassionate to ourselves as we get through these murky waters. We also need to be compassionate to the fatigue that might be setting in around us, as sometimes our carers and loved ones need extra support or professional help too.

In the year after cancer, fatigue had set in with some around me and what had been more positive language had become less positive and even critical. Not long after finishing my initial treatment, it had come back to me that someone had said, *"She just needs to get over it (cancer). She has too much time on her hands to think about it."* Bearing in mind that this was said not long after my BRCA1 mutation diagnosis whilst I was also coping with the longer term treatment changes, it's not surprising that I may have still had a bit to "get over." Sometimes when comments like this come back to us, we need to be able to pick our battles, which might mean just letting them go and moving on, but at other times, we need to confront people and explain the realities that we are in. It's easier for others to be compassionate to us and soften their stance when they afford us the courtesy of listening.

Surrounding Yourself with Supporters

Even for those of us who are lucky enough to have a support network as we move through the cancer pathway, it's not uncommon to lose confidence and self-worth, particularly when our cancers affect our working and home life abilities and capacities, thus bringing a drop in our performance. Climbing out of the cancer space of disadvantage and disempowerment can be helped tremendously, when people in our networks amplify us and speak up for us. I found it so therapeutic when others placed value on me, because sometimes, it just wasn't going to come from within.

One such time that comes to mind was when I experienced a few unexpected blank cognitive and memory moments courtesy of menopause and chemotherapy during a fairly high powered meeting back in 2007. Seeing the shock, panic and vulnerability rising within me, a colleague and friend covered for me, and spoke on my behalf in a way that seemed natural and even pre-planned. She helped me maintain my dignity and created a safe space for me, despite my somewhat embarrassing moment. It made me realize how important it is, particularly when vulnerable, to make sure that you have supportive people alongside you who will bat for you, even if the going gets tough. My friend's action was a perfect example of genuine compassion and support, and when going through cancer, it is very true to say that we need nothing less.

Mindset and How to Help Yourself

"You gain strength, courage, and confidence by every experience in which you really stop to look fear in the face...You must do the thing you think you cannot do."

Eleanor Roosevelt's quotation really struck a chord. I couldn't always change my circumstances, but I could look my fears in the face and take action to put my life in order, even when it was hard, and even when it felt like it was beyond me.

I would try to consciously think about what I wanted to achieve in the future, so that when opportunities came my way, I would be ready for them. Remaining forward thinking was also therapy in itself. It spurred me on to do more and be more, and helped me to get out of my own way, forgetting about the day-by-day discomfort and minutae of details of my cancer pathway. In it's place, it had me thinking more about the big picture and the more important things in life, like my purpose, undertaking meaningful work and projects, and enjoying my time with family and friends.

I also often found strength and courage when I looked at the example that others had set who had walked this path before me. So many women and men (including my ancestors) had so bravely looked fear in the face, to pave the way so that women like me could now have a better chance of survival and be able to live with a better quality of life compared to days gone by. Their stories were inspiring, and they had also shown us that life could be good again, if we were prepared to face our adversities, and do the work.

When You Need Psychological Help, Get It!

Friends, family and others in the community can only offer so much when it comes to psychological support during the cancer experience, even if they're truly amazing. I've met people who have been essentially stuck in an intensely self-focused cycle whereby they perseverate on their cancer stories week after week, without a shift, change or resolution. These folks have often been reticent to seek help and I've seen them struggle, and their relationships suffer. The services that counsellors and psychologists provide are vital. It's easy for all of us to get stuck in a rut, but it really is important that we get professional help before things become catastrophic, or before mental health or relationships decline. It's also important to get help not only to get through, but also to help us to get the most out of life.

There is always someone out there who is just the one for us and can help us on our way. Sometimes, we need to have the courage to put up our hands to ask for help, and sometimes we need to do a little bit of work to find the person who is right for us. When we do, it can be one of the best investments in both time and energy that we can ever make.

The Work of Dr. Brené Brown

"Empathy has no script. There is no right way or wrong way to do it. It's simply listening, holding space, withholding judgement, emotionally connecting, and communicating that incredibly healing message that you're not alone."

—Brené Brown.

Cancer is messy. We all need to be prepared to learn and grow together when having tough and honest conversations, and be ok that we will get it both right and wrong.

I'll leave you with some ideas about empathy thanks to the fantastic work of Dr. Brené Brown from Texas, USA. I've found her work so helpful and have really enjoyed deepening my understanding not only on empathy, but also on vulnerability and emotional intelligence. I wish that I had access to her work at the time of my diagnosis.

Dr. Brown (2020) explains that empathy occurs in four stages, including:

1. **Perspective Taking** or putting yourself in someone else's shoes.
2. **Staying out of Judgement** and listening.
3. **Recognizing Emotion** in another person that you may have felt before.
4. **Communicating** that you can recognize that emotion.

My experience is that many of us find all the stages somewhat difficult, but having the courage to communicate that we've recognized an emotion is probably the hardest stage, and the one that we don't naturally think to do. To me, this doesn't need to always be conveyed verbally. I've been in the company of many who let me know that they've recognised my emotion without saying a word, but have rather communicated the message of *"I see you, I've heard you, and I get it."* This has further opened the door to deeper connections and relationships with those around me, and has reduced any feelings of isolation that I have had. Empathy can be so healing.

Conclusion

As people who've had cancer, we need to contend with the strains and discomfort that cancer-related vulnerability and disadvantage can bring. However, we are always in a position to have some influence over our circumstances, and can help others to help us. We need to be prepared to speak up, educate others and even call others out when appropriate. Developing empathy, high emotional intelligence and the language to express emotions takes time after cancer. But it is a critical step to ultimately help us heal and bring us together. Connecting meaningfully and even deeply with those around us is what life is about, after all.

"We don't have to do all of it alone"
(Brown, 2020).

10.

Cancer Therapies.
Strengths And
Imperfections.

———•———

*"Health is about so much more than simply
not being sick. It's about getting a balance
between physical, mental, emotional, cultural
and spiritual health."*
**—Dr. Tamara MacKean, Aboriginal Waljen
Woman, Western Australia**

E ntering the cancer experience after having spent ten
years working in the health care sector gave me a unique

perspective to see the good things about the system and the physiotherapy profession, as well as the not so good. As I returned to the physio coalface after treatment, I realised that no matter which specialty area I worked in, if I was to continue to deliver care, I would need to be ok seeing people face adversity, confront losses and deal with the changes that their poor health had inflicted, just as I needed to do in my personal life. I felt that if I continued with the mindset that I'd established during my training and career thus far, and focus on my role and purpose as a physiotherapist to help and serve, I'd cope as I always had. And that would prove to be true.

Seeing the massive benefits and power that allied health services had in the oncology space and having experienced a marked lack of it, I decided to help fill the gap and established a private physiotherapy service which came to be known as Breast, Gynae, and Lymph (BGAL) Physiotherapy. Being self-employed in the earlier years gave me the flexibility I needed to accommodate the surgeries that I still had ahead of me. Establishing the practice also felt like a win-win, by doing something that would make a difference, but would also be personally meaningful and positive.

My aim with setting up the practice was to provide an integrated and holistic physio service, caring for people during and after surgery, chemo and radiation therapy. Our services could address many side effects of treatment, including scar tissue management, pain, cardio-respiratory and muscular deconditioning, impaired movement and flexibility, lymphoedema, menopause issues, and pelvic floor/sexual health concerns. I also saw the potential it had to expand into other allied health services, including dietetics and exercise physiology.

My Therapeutic Journey

In retrospect, I would have preferred to receive more information prior to my surgery about cording, seromas and also the medium and longer term goals with my recovery. I'd only had one short physiotherapy consultation by the bedside that had consisted of teaching me early exercises to do after the surgery, so it hadn't been as informative or empowering as I felt it needed to be. To rehabilitate after my initial breast surgery, one health care professional even said, *"Just do your ADLs (or activities of daily living). That will be all you need."* It made me realize how little some in the health fraternity understood about the impacts of treatment side effects and their patient's needs in their everyday lives. My normal day to day activities involved distance swimming and doing heavy patient handling, so how my ADLs were going to provide the stepping stones to help me return to them, I didn't know! I had more questions than answers, few guidelines to work with, and a relatively small amount of research to base my rehabilitation on in those earlier days.

In 2007, there had also been conflicting information about lymph node care with some health professionals recommending the avoidance of arm activity on the operated side to run the risk of causing an onset or increasing existing lymphoedema or swelling of the arm or chest. I found it bizarre that virtually all areas of health otherwise encouraged exercise, yet with lymph care there seemed to be a totally different set of rules. Thankfully, my treating team weren't subscribers to this bizarre theory even though some of their colleagues were still recommending it. I also found that the available information on lymphoedema was generic, and didn't give me specific details about my individual sitation, what was safe to do, nor about what outcomes I should expect.

How I Got Started

I was keen to be part of raising the bar for how, when, and what we offered as physios, knowing first-hand that we could offer so much to help get people back on track. Until my diagnosis, only a small number of people around Australia, and indeed the world, had championed breast or general oncology physiotherapy, with a larger, but still modest number of practitioners specialised in lymphoedema therapy. A few therapists had worked very hard and had advocated for increased breast, lymph and oncology physiotherapy service provision, but nevertheless, it seemed remarkable that there were still so few practitioners when cancer affected so many.

I started the ball rolling by enrolling in my Master of Clinical Physiotherapy, majoring in women's health in 2009. The course enabled me to learn more about many facets of women's health, from cancer therapies, exercise and rehabilitation, to lymphoedema, pelvic and sexual health, bone health and menopausal health. My enrolment not only gave me some sense of moving forward when I felt like I was being held back, but it also directly gave me more skills to rehabilitate and recover personally.

I soon added other qualifications, including lymphoedema accreditation (basic and advanced) and a pilates diploma (Polestar), which helped me to be able to provide a more holistic physio and exercise service over the cancer continuum. The pilates training proved to be instrumental in particular for my rehabilitation after my initial breast and reconstruction surgeries, and my gynae surgery. The variability of exercises with the focus on movement quality, control, stability and form, allowed for more sophisticated, real life movement patterns, which I felt was particularly good for my shoulder girdle, core and pelvic floor function. Some studies have since shown positive effects of pilates after breast cancer treatment also (Boing et al., 2020; Stan et al., 2012), and when done well, it's benefits to pelvic floor control and health (Culligan et al., 2010; Coleman et al., 2015).

It was a bit of a job to get BGAL off the ground, but within a few years referrals were on a roll and the practice started to build a good reputation for delivering good care. The next challenge as it grew however, was to find someone to join me. Even though there was now more awareness of the significant value that allied health professions (such as physio, occupational therapy, dietetics and exercise physiology) could add to the cancer space, the lack of access to training opportunities and inadequate funding of our services had been conducive to workforce shortages. I managed to get through the load by working long hours, but at times, not getting the time out that I would have preferred was a bit intense. By 2016, I finally found a perfect women's health physiotherapist to join me, and helped train her in breast physiotherapy (given the lack of breast physiotherapy training pathways). It was great having her on board, being both passionate about the specialty, and possessing wonderful physio and interpersonal skills.

Now at over 12 years since establishment, the practice has continued to go from strength to strength. The BGAL team has now cared for almost 4000 people diagnosed with breast and gynae cancer, melanoma and prostate cancer. From having started as a sole trader, we now have a team of six. It has been really pleasing that we've been able to offer an individualised responsive service, with both scope and difference. However, there has not been time to rest on our laurels, with us still working hard to keep on top of our game, and meet the variety of needs of all who come to see us.

Sadly however, by in large, our public and private funding in oncology continues to assume that our therapy is no different from any other specialty area. The funding of interventions are therefore benchmarked with clinical areas that only require short term and brief consultations (for example, with those required to treat mild pain or simple rehabilitation after a basic surgical procedure). This transferred funding model into oncology has remarkably undercut what is needed to treat the whole body and the whole person, particularly after the complex and compounding treatments and conditions that invariably come with a diagnosis (i.e. post surgical and lymphoedema management, exercise during/ after chemotherapy, rehabilitation from reconstruction etc.). Along with our colleagues around the globe, we continue to lobby the government and other funding bodies to try to improve allied health funding, but as yet in Australia, no changes have materialised.

The Power of Allied Health Interventions

It has been really exciting seeing where the research in oncology physiotherapy has been going since my diagnosis. Research has shown numerous benefits in physiotherapy breast cancer care, reducing lymphoedema, pain and fatigue, and improving shoulder range, physical function, overall quality of life and psychological wellbeing (Olsson Möller et al., 2019; Lacomba et al., 2009; McNeely et al., 2012; De Groef et al., 2015). In Australia, lymphoedema care is now recommended to be part of the standard of care for breast surgery with nodal removal (Cancer Australia, 2020). However, unfortunately in most cases, lymph care still seems to remain ad hoc for those who've had skin, gynaecologic or prostate cancer related lymph node removal.

Research looking at the benefits of exercise during and after treatment has also come into its own. I knew of the early proven benefits of exercise after cancer and formally added it into my survivorship action plan back in 2007, however the evidence has continued to become clearer and even more compelling over the last 10 to 15 years. Exercise has been shown to minimise treatment's side effects, improve recovery and even improve survival. With breast cancer, exercising to a moderate level (150 mins of moderate-intensity cardio per week) has shown a reduction in recurrence risk by 30 to 50% (Friedenreich et al., 2019; Irwin et al., 2008; Holmes et al., 2005). These benefits are thought to be due to exercise stimulating natural killer cells (a type of immune cell), modifying hormones like oestrogen and reducing carcinogenic activity (Friedenreich et al., 2017). There may also be benefits to exercising around the time of chemotherapy infusion as exercise has been shown to increase the delivery of the therapy to tumour sites, increasing its efficacy (Schadler et al., 2016).

Exercise can also reduce a number of side effects from treatment, including fatigue, nausea and psychological distress, and can also improve fitness, muscle strength, functional ability and quality of life (Clinical Oncology Society of Australia, 2018). Consequently, the Clinical Oncology Society of Australia recommends that exercise interventions are integrated into the cancer care pathway, standing alongside chemo and radiation as standard care. There is also evidence that higher physical activity levels may prevent some cancers from occurring in the first place, including breast, bowel and prostate cancers (Friedenreich et al., 2019; Hayes et al., 2009). So, my advice would be, if you're not yet moving, get to it, as the evidence is becoming compelling!

Lymphatic Developments

Our understanding of the lymphatic system has also come along in leaps and bounds since I started my lymphatic studies in 2009. People are also no longer encouraged to avoid using their arms after nodal removal, as exercise studies clearly show that a graduated and mixed exercise program does not cause an onset of lymphoedema or worsen lymphoedema symptoms (Schmitz et al., 2010). It is also known that if people are leaner with less fatty weight, this can also significantly reduce the risk of developing lymphoedema and can reduce its severity if established (Struiver et al., 2015).

A new lymphatic imaging technology using a dye called indocyanine green, has also helped us learn more about lymphatic anatomy and physiology, and will allow for a personalised approach to manual lymphatic drainage (Suami et al., 2019). This imaging has also enabled therapists to develop more effective massage techniques to further improve drainage efficacy (J.P. Belgrado, personal communication, May 5, 2017). So in time, we hope to see further reductions in lymphoedema severity and prevalence, given these lifestyle and exercise findings, alongside the lymphatic imaging and treatment advances.

Reconstruction Considerations

Over the last 14 years, one area that I haven't seen as much progress as I would have liked from a decision making and follow up care perspective, is in breast reconstruction. I'm not sure that reconstruction types are always tailored to the patients' needs and preferences, and I also question whether people are able to access rehabilitation services with appropriate professionals who understand their unique needs. Some reconstructive surgeons still have a notion that reconstructing the breast using muscle tissue from donor sites, such as the latissimus dorsi or TRAM, does not affect arm or abdominal function respectively. I have often been curious to know if these reconstructive procedures had been done on a man, whether we would even begin to entertain this notion! I get that many have worked hard to be able to give us back some dignity using these sophisticated and clever procedures, but it's equally important to give the facts and let women decide on what will work best for them.

It doesn't help when research appears to be unclear on the issue either. When I look at latissimus research, some research does suggest that strength and functional losses do exist (Sowa et al., 2016; Forthomme et al., 2010), but that these changes are virtually undetectable once recovery has occurred six months to a year down the track (Smith, 2014). Unfortunately, when I've looked closer at the latissimus studies that haven't noted change, however, from a physiotherapy viewpoint, I have noticed flaws in their methodology.

One flaw is that the measurement tools that have been used are often not adequately sensitive to detect the changes or losses experienced by the latissimus reconstruction once recovered (i.e. holding a pen, or playing cards is very unlikely to be affected). So, aspects that will more noticeably be effected, such as shoulder stability on load (i.e. planks), muscle endurance (i.e. long distance swimming) and higher level strength tasks (i.e. lifting heavier weights), will rarely be included in many measurement tools used. Subjective reporting can also be unreliable, as some people will have low levels of physical activity that will not necessarily detect changes that would be of significance to others undergoing the procedure with higher levels of activity. So, methodological variations, along with other confounding factors, can contribute to muddying the waters (Smith, 2014).

Therefore, the most important thing when considering breast reconstruction is to have all the facts at hand, especially given that the supporting research still remains relatively limited. My advice would be to speak to women who've had the surgery you are considering, have similar lifestyles, and have similar levels of physical activity, and hear their perspective. It may also sometimes be worth seeking a second opinion before signing up for breast surgery or reconstruction. All surgical options have their imperfections, including mastectomies without reconstructions, but you just want to know what they are. Just remember too that your medical situation may dictate what kind of surgery or reconstruction is going to be appropriate for you, as not all women will have all options available to them.

It's Never too Late to Heal, But Timing Does Matter

A few years back, I was referred to see an 80-year-old lady who had been diagnosed with breast cancer some forty years earlier, when there was little attention to survivorship care, nor access to allied health services. She had been a medical specialist herself and had had a mastectomy, lymph node clearance and radiation. She had lost considerable arm movement from the contracted radiation fibrosis or scar tissue, which did little for her arm function, comfort levels or lymphoedema.

At no time over those 40 years since her diagnosis, did any health professional think to refer her onto physiotherapy until, fortunately, she had been talking to a colleague of ours who knew about our work. We did much release work on the scar tissue, and implemented a number of strategies to minimise her lymphoedema and increase her range of shoulder and chest movement. Her function, freedom of movement, and heaviness of her arm improved within a few sessions, and even to this day, she continues to attend the practice for "top-up" therapy sessions. For me personally, it showed how adaptable tissues could still be, and how much of a difference therapy could still make so many years following her treatment.

The message from her story and those of others though, is that referrals to allied health services need to be part and parcel with breast cancer care and they need to be timely. Otherwise we may see unnecessary issues that arise down the track and less than ideal recovery, reducing these people's potential outcomes and adding to their discomfort and struggle. It is always so sad for those of us who are in the know, that ladies like my patient, have had to live with post-treatment issues for so long, not knowing that something could be done. In particular, lymphoedema can be very unforgiving once its inflammatory cycle has started. When beyond mild in severity also, it can be very hard to reverse. The establishment of a limited range of motion and altered movement patterns can also add stresses and strains to the tissues, increasing the prevalence of things down the track like shoulder impingement, costochondritis, middle back and neck pain, etc. (Lauridsen et al., 2008; McNeely et al., 2012). So, early and timely referrals are not an option. They are imperative.

Oncology Care is a Team Effort

I have been pleased that over recent years, with the professional support from our colleagues such as breast, gynae and reconstructive surgeons and cancer nurses, patients are being referred to see us earlier and routinely, as part of their cancer care. Our referrers understand the importance of patients knowing what to expect from surgery, what they can do to help their recovery, what they need to avoid for the time being, and the exercises and stretches to help them get there. They also understand that to manage lymphoedema or lymphoedema risk, people need to learn about the lymphatic system: what it is, how it works, what can go wrong after surgery, how they can optimise lymph care, and what to do should they develop the symptoms of lymphoedema (i.e. swelling, discomfort and heaviness).

The BGAL team has also really enjoyed working being a key contributor to cancer care alongside the multi-disciplinary oncology teams at St John of God Hospital (SJOG) in Subiaco (including the teams at Perth Specialist Breast Care, Western Australian Gynae and Surgery, and Genesis Cancer Care). We have really enjoyed the fact that they are not only excellent practitioners, but that they are patient-focused, collaborative and think holistically about people's care needs. It has also been great being recognised for our unique skills and contribution to the patient pathway, as well as being part of the positive culture that values compassion and innovation. Having worked in many workplaces over the years and having been a patient in a number too, I know that this isn't always the way that it goes.

Food and Nutrition

The research on diet and cancer is a work in progress (Cancer Council NSW, 2020). However, the more I read, the more I think that good nutrition is a form of cancer medicine, just as exercise is deemed to be. Attention to diet can be of value to help manage our weight, bowel health and overall health, and may even potentially reduce our risk of recurrence, including after a diagnosis of breast cancer (Ee et al., 2020).

Current research supports healthy eating habits, such as eating less red meat and processed foods, balancing fatty acids, and eating more fermented foods, whole foods and fibre (Taschery, 2014). Nutrients found in fruit and vegetables may also help to lower the risk of cancer, particularly those containing protective components such as vitamins, minerals, antioxidants and phytochemicals (like carotenoids, flavonoids, and isoflavonoids). However, the evidence to support this remains limited at this stage (Cancer Council NSW, 2020). We also know that alcohol avoidance can reduce the risk of both cancer development and recurrence in some cancers, including breast cancer.

So, we have only seen the tip of the iceberg regarding diet in the oncology space, but it's worth learning more about the value of nutrition in the context of cancer, and worth considering whether a consultation with a dietician might be beneficial.

The Power of Complementary Therapy

Having lived the cancer experience, I've come to understand firsthand that Complementary and Alternative Medicines (CAMS) can be very helpful for many people diagnosed with cancer. For me also, many of the CAMS modalities made sense to add to my traditional medical care, as they often complimented my understanding of health and wellness as a physiotherapist. I particularly benefitted from therapies based on some eastern philosophies, such as the Chakra system used in yoga and the

Chinese Meridian system used for traditional acupuncture therapies. CAMS research has also shown some promising results and many positive patient-reported outcomes, particularly relating to acupuncture, massage and yoga.

Acupuncture research has shown a reduction in chemotherapy-related nausea and vomiting, and suggests that it may also reduce anxiety, fatigue, hot flushes, and some types of pain (Cancer Council NSW, 2020). Similarly, massage has also gained more evidence base, showing effective reductions in pain, anxiety, depression, nausea, and fatigue in people who have had chemotherapy or surgery for cancer (Cancer Council NSW, 2020).

Yoga studies have demonstrated evidence of beneficial effects on psychological, physical and emotional health, and quality of life after a cancer diagnosis. It has also been noted, that yoga may enrich some patients' spiritual needs that are not met by conventional therapy, thereby further increasing overall wellness and well-being (Agarwal & Maroko-Afek, 2018). Many other medicines, such as Qi Gong, and mind-body medicines (including meditation, relaxation, art therapy, music, dance, cognitive therapy, etc.), are also reported to be beneficial by many people who walk the cancer path, so they are well worth investigation.

Studies have even shown that basic human touch including hugging, holding hands and even patting a furry friend can reduce stress. They can also increase feel-good chemicals such as oxytocin and serotonin to further improve one's ability to handle conflict, and improve relationships when facing health issues (Burge, 2019). Trust and connection developed between treating health care professionals, partners and the patient cannot be underestimated either. We know that people have higher survival when they get on with and like their treating practitioners (Alessy et al., 2019) and when they are married or in a partnership (Gomez, 2016). I've also found that therapy can provide an invaluable opportunity for patients to be chaperoned and coached through the cancer pathway, helping them to re-integrate after their treatments, both physically and mentally.

Conclusion

The power of cancer treatments and therapies is coming into its own thanks to many working both behind the scenes and at the coalface in health services and research. Accessing allied health services and holistic and integrated cancer care services, alongside choosing good lifestyle habits and self-care practices, provides a comprehensive way to get the best possible healing and recovery after a cancer diagnosis. Research is a big part of this shift and continues to propel us forward into a better tomorrow.

11.

A Better Tomorrow. Research Making A Difference.

"Do the best that you can until you know better. Then when you know better, do better."

—Maya Angelou.

Over many decades, experiencing breast and ovarian cancer has made us very aware of the progress made from research, and what it has meant for both us as a family and others. So much passion, time and expertise have gone into countless research trials to make tomorrow better. Although treatment improvements continue to emerge, they never seem to happen fast enough when either ourselves or our loved ones are in the hot seat. Such is the challenge of cancer—if only what will be discovered tomorrow was available today!

The Early Days

With little to no diagnostic or treatment prowess in the world of cancer at the time, very little had been available to my ancestors, the two Charlottes, except in my grandmother's case, some basic surgery and a soon to be discontinued microwave treatment via the Tronado machine. But time moved on in the cancer space, particularly in the 1980s by the time of my aunt's diagnosis in 1984. There was beginning to be an understanding that cancer risks could be inherited via genetic mutations with my aunt's medical oncologist, Dr. Trotter, stating that he was certain there was a genetic link of Merrel's breast cancer to my grandmother's ovarian cancer but that, *"We just don't know what it is yet."*

The 1980s and Onwards

Breast and Reconstructive Surgery

Merrel had gone straight to having a mastectomy and axillary clearance, because the understanding at the time was that the entire breast was diseased, not just a potential part of it as we know today. By the time of my diagnosis in 2007, there was the option for women with more defined or smaller tumours to have breast conservation surgery, such as a lumpectomy, whereby only the affected part of the breast was removed. Obviously, this reduced a number of potential issues experienced by women, particularly when it came to things like scar tissue formation, altered body image and feelings of a loss of femininity. By 2007 also, if there was no obvious lymph node involvement when diagnosed, a sentinel node biopsy could be performed, whereby a small number of lymph nodes could be sampled. This less invasive technique came with fewer side effects like reduced pain, movement impairment and lymphoedema, which significantly improved care for many women.

Since Merrel's latissimus reconstructive surgery, we have seen the emergence of new procedures using tissue/ fat from the abdomen, buttocks and upper thigh areas, as well as the advent of a new reconstructive material called the acellular dermal matrix. DIEP reconstructions using fat from the abdomen are now more commonly seen, and we have also recently seen the emergence of the PAP flap (using tissue or fat from the upper thighs). I certainly would have qualified for the PAP flap if it had been around when I was diagnosed, and would have loved to have had that option given my physical activities such as swimming and yoga. Instead, I enjoy the fact that advancements like these will be available for others who come after me—just as it was for me. Such is the cycle of making a better tomorrow.

AirXpander® technology has also been introduced since my reconstruction in 2008, for the latissimus reconstruction procedure. The tissues are stretched to make room for the breast implant using air rather than saline. This technology reduces trips to the surgeons rooms for implant expansion, and can also reduce the time required between the two surgeries to six weeks or so (from six months). The lat dorsi procedure in some circumstances can now also be done using the *"scarless"* technique, whereby surgeons avoid the incision on the back and rather perform the whole procedure through an incision on the front of the chest wall. This procedure reduces the visual reminder of surgery that scars can give us, and can also help some women feel more comfortable wearing bathers, and strapless or low cut shirts and dresses.

I've also been really pleased seeing the emergence of oncoplastic surgeons since my diagnosis. These surgeons not only remove cancers, but they can also simultaneously perform a variety of reconstructions, preventing the need for women to have to wait for reconstruction down the track with two surgeons, as I needed to do. The reduction in the number of surgeries needed can make such a big difference on so many levels, reducing interruptions professionally, socially and financially, and eliminating the need for more recovery time.

Surgeons are also currently looking further into other options, such as pre-pectoral reconstructions, whereby breast implants sit in front of the pectoral muscles. These reconstructions use the newer acellular dermal matrices, and require little to no interruption to muscular tissue compared to other reconstructions. If this continues to be successful, this option is likely to be a real plus for many women diagnosed with breast cancer going forward, although as always, these reconstructions won't be appropriate for everyone, such as for those who've had radiation.

BRCA1 Trials and Progress

In 1994, ten years after Merrel was diagnosed with breast cancer, the BRCA1 gene was identified by Mary-Claire King and her team. Even since my testing 13 years later in 2007, it has been amazing seeing the huge leaps that technology can now deliver. Now my diagnosis alone would have enabled me to access testing, reducing the need to spend time prior to testing obtaining the necessary death certificate and medical records clearance. Testing can also now be performed during chemotherapy (it previously had to be done before or after chemotherapy), and can also be completed in two to three weeks rather than the months that I was told that it was going to take. The current fast turn-around of results therefore, can enable women to base some of their treatment decisions according to their genetic findings, such as undertaking immediate mastectomies and reconstructions for their initial surgery, rather than having to have this surgery later down the track (like my predecessors and I had).

Funded breast screening using MRIs for high-risk women (including for those with BRCA1) were also introduced in 2007, about six months after my diagnosis. With this more sensitive technology available for regular screening in Australia, breast cancers are more likely to be diagnosed at an earlier stage, hence improving women's prognoses.

An organisation that I've been involved with, called the Breast Cancer Trials Group (BCTG), was founded in 1978 when I was three. Over the years, they have undertaken a number of studies that have helped many of us who have a high risk of developing breast cancer. More recently also, the BCTG have opened a new ground-breaking prevention trial specifically for BRCA1 mutation carriers, called BRCA-P. BRCA-P predicts that the use of a drug called Denosumab, traditionally used to help strengthen bones in osteoporotic women, will be able to prevent BRCA1 breast cancer (and maybe ovarian cancer). This trial holds hope for the next generation including my cousin Gem's children, potentially paving the way for another option to prevent cancers, or at least to buy some time to enable us to keep our breasts and ovaries when we need them.

The research finding relating to fertility and the BRCA1 gene mutation will also potentially help women to be able to plan ahead, as we know that healthy BRCA1 mutation carriers have a 25% lower fertility rate at 35 than women without the mutation of the same age (Phillips et al., 2016). We may therefore see some mutation carriers have children and/ or IVF procedures earlier than they might have done otherwise. So, these studies are real game changers, and will enable women to make informed decisions about family planning, and enable them to be a step ahead of, and outsmart these adverse consequences of BRCA1.

Medical Oncology

Some breast surgeons found it hard to get their heads around the idea in the 1970s and 80s, that in early breast cancer, chemotherapy could potentially mop up micro-metastatic disease and further improve survival. So at the time of Merrel's diagnosis, the paradigm shift had just occurred, Merrel found herself being one of the early ones off the block, seeing her undertake an early chemo regimen known as CMF.

In the years between our diagnoses, the regimes for triple-negative cancer would progress, seeing improved survival by adding an anthracycline chemotherapy, Adriamycin, and a taxane called Paclitaxel to the existing Cyclophosphamide agent. Around the time of my diagnosis also, the benefits of the two weekly dose-dense therapy treatments that I undertook (rather than three weekly treatments) were also coming to be known, hence Arlene, my medical oncologist's recommendation. So with these changes, it's not hard to understand some of the reasons why the overall survival rate at five years improved from 75% at the time of Merrel's diagnosis in 1984, to the current rate of 91% (Australian Institute of Health and Welfare, 2020). With more research and the addition of novel and groundbreaking treatments, this figure is likely to keep improving also.

If I was diagnosed today, it is likely that I would have been prescribed my chemotherapy before surgery (known as neoadjuvant chemotherapy), thus enabling the treatment of my cancer earlier, allowing for my genetic testing prior to surgery, therefore potentially reducing the number of surgeries that I may have needed by combining my reconstruction with the breast and axillary surgery. At the current time also, we are seeing potential treatment improvements with the emergence of immunotherapy trials in triple-negative breast cancer. We hope that the positive results of the immunotherapy trials in other cancers will now also translate across into the "triple-negative" space.

I hope too that research continues to demonstrate improvements in survival whilst also reducing the treatment-related toxicity that we've seen in times past. It is so important that we not only improve survival, but that we also get improved survival outcomes with a better quality of life, so that cancer survivors can continue to live well and thrive.

Radiation Therapy

Radiation therapy has seen changes over the years too. Having sustained a degree of cadiac injury after radiation, I've been really pleased to see the emergence of the deep inspiratory breath-holding technique when delivering radiation over the left chest wall. This will mean that going forward, women will be spared the collateral damage to adjacent tissues that older radiation techniques contributed to.

Radiation can now also be delivered when appropriate over a shorter three-week period rather than five or six weeks. It can even now also be delivered intra-operatively at the time of surgery for some women, avoiding the daily radiation treatments needed with external beam therapy. For some, daily treatments can significantly impact people's lives, especially when people are working or living in rural and remote areas, so advances such as these can make such a big difference. Radiation therapy has also more recently shown additional reductions in tumour growth, not only in the field of therapy but also elsewhere in the body using what is known as the abscopal effect (Yilmaz et al., 2019). This is a very exciting development and may offer a clue in how we can further treat metastatic disease in the years ahead.

The Future

When it comes to cancer, three big questions still remain for researchers. The first one is, how can we prevent all cancers from occurring in the first place? There will no doubt be a multitude of answers to this complex question, given the huge diversity and variability of different cancers. The second question will be, which cancers will really benefit from particular treatments such as chemotherapy and radiation? The better we get at answering these questions, the better we can allocate the resources to treat those people who really need it, and are going to respond to it. The third one is, for those diagnosed with cancer, how can we stop tumours from metastasizing? If we can find the key to this lock, we will be one big step closer to saving more lives.

MY STORY

The Present and The Future.

—•————————————————•—

12.

The Power Of Tomorrow. A Story Of Hope, Love And Connection.

———•————————•———

"Memories are the key, not to the past, but to the future."

—Corrie Ten Boom

Like many, I thought that the main job of overcoming early-stage breast cancer would be the things that are well known, such as overcoming losing my breasts and hair, and tolerating

the short-term side effects of chemotherapy. But there were so
many other factors to be confronted and managed in the quest
to survive and have at least some quality of life. The bumps in
the road and unexpected findings presented for a number of
years also, showing that even with an early cancer diagnosis
that proved to be curable, it could still be quite a marathon to
get through and turn things around.

My Present

When I reflect, I am ok with the decisions that I've made
along the way regarding my cancer and BRCA1 management.
It has been about choosing the lesser of all evils and finding
the strength and courage to keep moving forward towards a
better tomorrow. Sure, it would have been great if PAP flap
breast reconstructions and the deep inspiratory breath-hold
technique had been available when I had my reconstruction
and radiotherapy respectively, but as with anyone who walks
this path, we can only work with the best that science and
technology can offer us at each point in time. And fortunately
for me, the treatments proved to be enough to see me through,
and for that, I have been incredibly grateful.

I've heard some people say that it has been a privilege to have had
cancer. I can't say that the word privilege resonates with me in
any way, but I've learned a lot through my personal experience
and the experiences of my family, so hopefully I've come to be
a better person for it. It has also made me realise how special
my family, friends and a number of cancer organizations are.
They have helped me immeasurably, not only to re-integrate

as a person, but also to thrive post-diagnosis. I am also forever grateful to my medical team who walked with me along the path; my two breast surgeons, medical oncologist, radiation oncologist, gynae oncologist, reconstructive surgeon, fertility specialist, menopausal gynaecologist, clinical geneticist, cardiologist, gastroenterologist and the numerous nurses, therapists, counsellors, and other health care personnel who have helped me through. Without all of them, I wouldn't have made it through as well as I have, if at all.

Now 14 years later, I continue to juggle a few ongoing sequelae of my diagnosis and treatments. I currently have annual breast ultrasounds as there have been some issues with textured implants causing a rare cancer called ALCL in a very small number of women. So, given that my implants need to be exchanged in a few years time, I will change them to smooth implants to avoid the hassle of having to be monitored so closely. Despite this hiccup though, I'm still glad and thankful that I've had the opportunity to have reconstruction, and that is has allowed me to visually keep me, being me. From a post-oopherectomy perspective, I continue to keep an eye on my HRT as it sometimes needs some adjusting to keep on top of things. I also continue to have bone density scans every two years given my premature menopause, and so far so good. Women's hormonal changes from breast cancer can certainly make us a more complex and trickier nut to crack, that's for sure!

From a movement and lymphoedema point of view, I have managed to maintain full chest and shoulder mobility despite the tissue tightening from the radiation treatment over the years. From time to time, I also experience low-grade transient arm lymphoedema. Thankfully I've managed to keep it at bay, due to good underlying lymphatic function, good body awareness, and good access and skills to manage my lymphatic care. I also intermittently wear my compression sleeve when I feel or see a backlog of fluid collecting particularly in my upper arm. I find that a flexible and early approach of management off loads my lymphatics when it needs it, and helps me to nip it in the bud.

I continue to find that exercising keeps me in good shape both mentally and physically, especially when I'm outdoors in nature, fresh air and the gentle sun. I still exercise regularly, continuing with my open water distance swimming, as well as my walking, cycling, yoga and pilates. Some yoga positions remain difficult, especially the ones with high upper body load, endurance and stability needs. So, I keep everything as good as I can, including my core and lower body function, and modify yoga postures and activities as needed. I'm a tad more used to the loss of my top fitness level cardiac wise, but I still need to confront this frustration from time to time. My main aim for now, is to keep things as good as possible for as long as possible, and to remain grateful, given that many others have not been so lucky.

In relation to cancer genetics, it has been encouraging to see more developments in the recent past from a support perspective, especially knowing how hard the road can be without these services. I've seen the development of BRCA networking events, support groups and social media groups, which can help to reduce the isolation, whilst also providing a platform for communication between people experiencing similar issues. I've also been pleased to see a shift towards increased medium and longer-term follow up care for those of us with cancer susceptibility genes, to address issues like menopausal management and family planning. However, at the current point of time, there are still unknowns into the best way to manage us, especially relating to infertility, weaning hormone replacement and managing overall health. It will be a work in progress for some time.

My Profession

My work life since my diagnosis has certainly been full and colourful, from having established BGAL, to teaching in the university setting, to joining forces with others in the profession to raise the awareness of the important contribution that we make. It has been exciting seeing the knowledge base grow, as well as meeting and learning from many extra-ordinary practitioners both from within Australia and abroad. What I would now like to see is the matching of funding for physiotherapy, lymph care, exercise and dietetics care to what we see in psychology. I still find it frustrating that in the main part, people can access more funding for psychological help to talk about their concerns about their lymphoedema and other adverse physical outcomes, than they are able to access the care to actually be able to do something about it. But such is the current state of cancer funding in Australia. I hope and feel, however, that the profile for allied health professions will now start to come into it's own, particularly on the back of consumer advocacy, the push for patient-centred care and also the compelling exercise research data.

My BGAL team has consisted of such wonderful high calibre colleagues, and it has been fantastic to see the love and care they put into their work and patients. For me personally, after 12 years of hands-on physiotherapy work in oncology, I decided to hang up my boots. I had known for a while that the time had come to leave the clinical coalface and step back. I achieved the things that I had really wanted to and now wanted more space away from the direct emotion and pain of cancer that although cushioned from to an extent, we still have to work with at the coalface. I'd cared for around 2000 people diagnosed with cancer, and felt in my heart of hearts that I'd done what I could. I now manage the practice and plan to branch out into other areas of interest, and look forward to seeing where allied health research and services progress to in the years to come.

Love Finally Came

True love did come to me and arrived a good nine years after diagnosis. The no-goes finally ended, and after having worked for a few months alongside the oncoplastic surgeons at Perth Specialist Breast Care, I took a stab and asked Lee out. I'd met him about three or four years prior at a breast nurses education day where we had both presented. I thought he was really nice and tried to speak to him after the event, but although I tried, I didn't manage to catch him. I'd also thought that as nice of a guy as he was, he was probably off the market anyway!

When it came to asking Lee out, I took the lead by asking myself around to his apartment to watch the annual Australia Day fireworks. I thought if he wasn't into me, I would get over it soon enough. Life can be too short anyway, nothing ventured, nothing gained! As fate would have it, there was another event the following weekend, again in front of Lee's apartment. So again I invited myself over, enjoying this time, a beautiful outdoor performance of the West Australian Opera. Needless to say that both nights were lovely, and we really enjoyed each other's company.

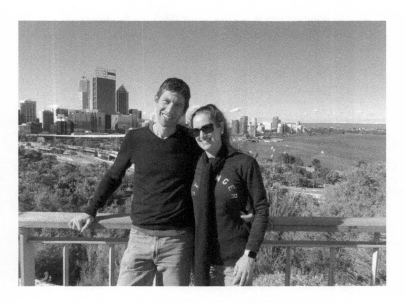

Lee and I overlooking Perth city.

Over the past few years, our relationship has been organic and has grown with a natural ease and flow. I guess we both did the hard yards in our own travels so that upon connecting, it could just happen without any major drama or issues. We love doing a lot of the same things as well, such as walking by the beach, travelling, swimming, and wining and dining. He allows me to just be me. I get meaning from being with him and I get perspective. There are no terms or conditions, just genuine friendship and honesty. Lee has also been able to hear me and understand me which has been really healing, but has also enabled him to get to know the real me.

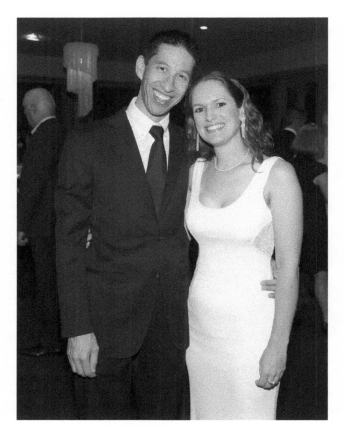

Lee and I at the St John of God Hospital Christmas Soiree © West Australian Newspapers Limited.

In relation to telling Lee about my cancer, I only ever had to say two things. One, that I was BRCA1 positive and also that I was diagnosed with breast cancer at 31 in 2007. He knew the rest from a medical and treatment viewpoint. It was such a change and a relief not to have to explain my situation, after having to do so over the prior eight years or so. Being so well informed about breast cancer also, Lee had no fears or reservations about my past, just knowledge and insight into what I've been through. I've been able to talk to him in my own way and my own time about the details, moment by moment and piece by piece, and I've felt like I've finally come home doing it. Now four years later, we are engaged. We both look forward to many happy times together.

Our Furry Family

After a few years into my relationship with Lee, our beautiful dog Ebony's time with us would come to an end. Her health took a turn for the worst in 2019 when she developed auto-immune anaemia, a condition where her body had started attacking her own red blood cells. She was on steroidal treatment which initially helped, but she progressively lost strength and was eventually unable to walk or control her bladder or bowel. Thankfully during her ill health, I was in a position to be able to nurse her and care for her, just as she had done for me all those years earlier. Things had now, however, come full circle, and our time together was about to come to an end. There was something, however, even beautiful about it. She had been such a big and important part of my life and had been with me the whole way. I think of her often.

Now, we have the next generation of fox terrier puppies who have something of Ebi's spirit in them. Billie and George are just as indefatigable and loving, and through them, we continue to learn about the rich tapestry of love that Ebi had so beautifully started.

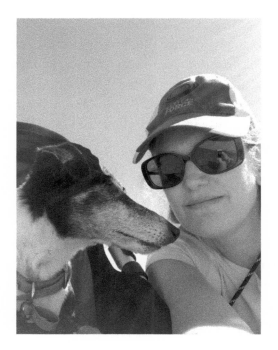

Ebi and I in her last weeks

In relation to my fertility, Lee and I talked at length about our options with the donor embryos offered by my incredible friends. But after much deliberation and thought, we both agreed that I had put in the best fight, and that it was time to accept our loss, and put my energy and passion elsewhere. The odds of success were low (I was told that making it to term when ovaries are no longer intact is about 5%), and my body had already gone through a lot. I'd seen people struggle with letting go of their hopes to have a family and I'd seen it destroy them, even when the writing was probably on the wall. I didn't want that for us. The truth was that my path of survival had come with some dreams being realized, and others not. Motherhood going forward for me, would need to come through our friends, nephews and nieces, as well as our new delightful furry family.

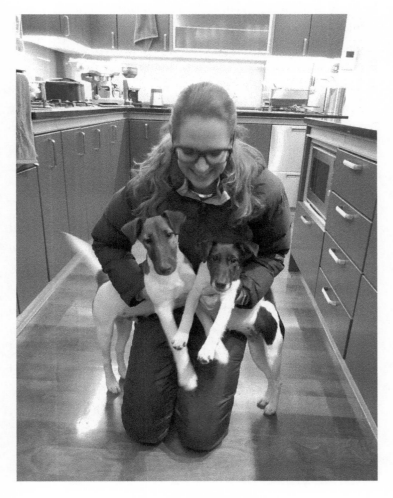

George, Billie and I

Memories of Friends and the Future for My Family

I think about my friends who have passed often and hold their memories in a special place. Joe, Cam, Jude and many others, have touched me so much, and I often wonder about what they would have been doing had they still been alive. I also often think about their families and loved ones. Since their passing, I can only imagine how hard it must be living through Christmases and birthdays and other special times. Joe, Cam and Jude also remind me to cherish as many memories as possible, and make me remember that life is a gift. Knowing that our lives also have a vicariousness about them, there is never a time like the present to make our lives all that we hope for, as much and as often as we can.

I often think of my grandmother and wonder what she would think about genetic testing and the technologies that we now have available. I'm glad that she never knew that we would also have to confront cancer just as she had. But, such is the way of genetic diseases. I hope that we can continue to find ways to outsmart it, or at least reduce the risks of getting cancer down considerably. My parents and siblings continue to thrive, and Ruby, my eldest niece, is now finishing school, driving a car and beginning university! Ashie, Alice and Lachie also continue to do well at school, as well as in their extra-curricular activities and sports.

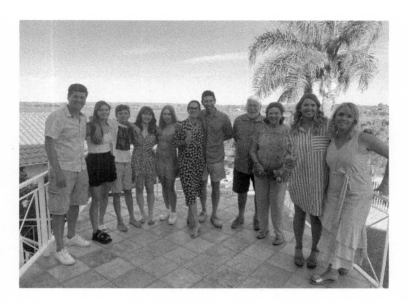

Burnett family celebrating our engagement

Merrel remains well, as is Gem. Gem has done so well to not only get through her cancer, but also to have overcome her drug challenges of the past. Together, we hope that her experience and pathway can encourage others to get through, even if it feels trying, hard, lonely and dark. We also keep our fingers and toes crossed that it goes ok for Gem's children when they come to have their genetic testing after they turn 18. We hope that as a family, should they be diagnosed with BRCA1, they can continue with the same strength and courage to navigate their paths that they have shown thus far. Ours hearts are with them.

It is at least of some comfort that the future of breast and ovarian cancer holds more promise than ever. Hopefully, through more preventative treatments, we can continue to prevent these cancers from occurring in the first place. We should also continue to see improved cancer diagnostics through the advent of more sophisticated and sensitive technologies, such as biomarker testing and improved imaging. I'm optimistic too, that we will continue to discover more tailored and effective treatments, and thus see improved survival and fewer side effects. I also hope that improved access to oncology allied health and integrated care services continues, so that people can enjoy a better quality of life and the return to holistic wellness and prosperity that they deserve.

My Conclusions

Since my diagnosis 14 years ago, I've gained a unique insight into so many aspects of life and the people in it. This has helped me to understand the wide ripple effects that ill health can have around us and also the numerous layers of challenges that can arise from just one diagnosis. I hope that by sharing my story and my friends' and family's stories, my book's title has more meaning, allowing for the breast cancer experience to be more comprehensively seen for what it is. It's not just about the breast; it's about so much more—context, change, uncertainty, loss, empathy, triumph and love, on many levels, and in so many ways.

Having lived through the twists and adversities of BRCA1, intergenerationally and round after round, and having experienced changes both visible and invisible, I feel like this chapter has finally closed and that a new one awaits. This chapter has come with some dreams being realized and others not, but this is the way that life can go at times. And although my courage has waxed and waned many times along the way, it has been a huge positive to be able to gather enough strength and somehow find my way back to wellness, happiness and prosperity. Even in my lowest moments when my reserves were low, tenacity and resolve would somehow emerge from deep within. At times this was thanks to the courage of my loving parents and my dear family and friends who'd stayed by me through thick and thin, helping me to find my way when things had got dark. At other times however, it had seemed to come from beyond the tangible. It was as though the love of my late ancestors had defiantly and unrelentingly spurred me on, lifting me up and propelling me forward— I just hadn't known or realised it for all that time.

I hope that you may find your peace, living your life with empathy, love and hope. I hope you surround yourself with people who support you and bring out the best in you. I hope you find deep healing through connecting with others, and find people who understand you and your world, giving you the dignity, compassion and respect that you need and deserve. Trust your wisdom and remain empowered, even when cancer may feel like it has taken your power and choices away from you. Get help when you need it, and keep your connections and relationships with others close and meaningful. Take action to make tomorrow better, even if today seems to elude you.

My story has been our story, past, present and future. *"Virescit Vulnere Virtus."* May courage grow strong at your wounds, always.

Postscript

———————●———————

If this book has brought up any issues, I urge you to get in touch with your treating medical specialists, general practitioner, allied health or nursing practitioner. If more personal in nature, ensure that you reach out to your friends, family, or support groups and services. It is so important to reach out to others who know your individual circumstances, your health system and you as a person.

References

Agarwal, R.P. & Maroko-Afek, A. (2018). Yoga into Cancer Care: A Review of the Evidence-based Research. *International Journal of Yoga, 11(1), 3–29.*

Alessy, A.A., Lüchtenborg, M. & Davies E.A. (2019). How have patient's experiences of cancer care been linked to survival? A systematic review. *Patient Experience Journal, 6(1): 63-80.*

American Cancer Society (2020). *Oncogenes and Tumour Suppressor Genes.* Retrieved from: https://www.cancer.org/cancer/cancer-causes/genetics/genes-and-cancer/oncogenes-tumor-suppressor-genes

Australian Institute of Health and Welfare & National Breast Cancer Centre (2006). *Breast cancer in Australia: an overview, 2006.* Cancer series no. 34. cat. no. CAN 29. Canberra: AIHW.

Boing, L., do Bem Fretta, T., de Carvalho Souza Vieira, M. et al. (2020). Pilates and dance to patients with breast cancer undergoing treatment: study protocol for a randomized clinical trial - MoveMama study. *Trials, 21(1):35.*

Brown, B. (2020). *How to have more empathy: Learn the four attributes of empathy from Brené Brown.* Retrieved from https://mrsmindfulness.com/four-attributes-of-empathy-brene-brown/

Burge, K. (2019). *Benefit of Human touch: What is the Impact on Our Health?* Retrieved from https://www.hcf.com.au/health-agenda/body-mind/mental-health/benefit-human-touch

Cancer Australia (2020). *Guidance for the management of early breast cancer: Recommendations and practice points.* Cancer Australia, Surry Hills, NSW.

Cancer Council Australia (2020). *Early Detection of Ovarian Cancer.* Retrieved from http://www.cancer.org.au/cancer-information/causes-and-prevention/early-detection-and-screening/early-detection-of-ovarian-cancer

Cancer Council NSW (2020). *Massage.* Retrieved from https://www.cancercouncil.com.au/cancer-information/living-well/complementary-therapies/body-based-practices/massage/

Cancer Council NSW (2020). *Nutrition and diet.* Retrieved from https://www.cancercouncil.com.au/cancer-prevention/diet-exercise/nutrition-and-diet/

Cancer Council NSW. (2020). *Other Paths to Parenthood.* Retrieved from https:www.cancercouncil.com.au/

cancer-information/managing-cancer-side-effects/
fertility-and-cancer/other-paths-to-parenthood

Cancer Council NSW. (2020). *Position statement – fruit, vegetables and cancer prevention*. Retrieved from https://wiki. cancer.org.au/policy /Position_ statement_Fruit,_vegetables_ and_cancer_prevention#Views_on_fruit_and_vegetables_in_ cancer_prevention_reports

Champ, N. (2020). *17 badass Brené Brown quotes that will inspire you to lead*. Retrieved from https: businesschicks. com/brene-brown-quotes/

Clinical Oncology Society of Australia. (2018). COSA Position Statement on Exercise in Cancer Care.

Coleman, T.J., Nygaard, I.E., Holder, D.N. et al. (2015). Intra-abdominal Pressure during Pilates: Unlikely to Cause Pelvic Floor Harm. *International Urogynecology Journal, 26(8): 1123–1130.*

Culligan, P.J., Scherer, J., Dyer, K. et al. (2010). A randomized clinical trial comparing pelvic floor muscle training to a Pilates exercise program for improving pelvic muscle strength. *International Urogynecology Journal, 21: 401–408.*

Cuzick, J., Sestak, I, Cawthorn, S. et al. (2015). Tamoxifen for prevention of breast cancer: extended long-term follow-up of the IBIS-I breast cancer prevention trial. *Lancet Oncology, 16: 67–75.*

De Groef, A., Van Kampen, M., Evi Dieltjens, E. et al. (2015). Effectiveness of Postoperative Physical Therapy for Upper-Limb Impairments After Breast Cancer Treatment: A systematic review. *Archives of Physical Medicine and Rehabilitation* 96 (6): 1140-1153.

Ee, C., Cave, A.E., Naidoo, D. et al. (2020). Weight before and after diagnosis of breast cancer or ductal carcinoma in situ: a national Australian survey. *BioMed Central Cancer,* 20: 113.

EVIQ (2020). *General practitioner referral guidelines for cancer genetics assessment.* Retrieved from https://www.eviq.org.au/p/1147

Fidler, M.M., Gupta, S., Soerjomataram, I., et al. (2017). Cancer incidence and mortality among young adults aged 20–39 years worldwide in 2012: a population-based study. *Lancet Oncology, 18: 1579–1589.*

Forthomme, B., Heymans, O., Jacquemin, D., et al. (2010). Shoulder function after latissimus dorsi transfer in breast reconstruction. *Clinical Physiology and Functional Imaging, 30: 406–412.*

Friedenreich, C.M., Stone, C.R., Cheung, W.Y. & Hayes, S.C. (2019). Physical Activity and Mortality in Cancer Survivors: A Systematic Review and Meta-Analysis. *JNCI Cancer Spectrum, 4(1): pkz080.*

Friedenreich, C.M., Shaw, E. & Heather K., Neilson, K. & Brenner, D.R. (2017). Epidemiology and biology of physical

References

activity and cancer recurrence. *Journal Molecular Medicine, 95(10): 1029-1041.*

Gomez, S.L. (2016). *Does marriage alone improve cancer survival? Taking a closer look.* Retrieved from https://scopeblog.stanford. edu/2016/05/09/does-marriage-alone-improve-cancer-survival-taking-a-closer-look/

Gurtin, Z. (2019). *Only 21% of women who use their frozen eggs become mothers.* Retrieved from https://medicalxpress.com/news/2019-05-women-frozen-eggs-mothers.html#

Hayes, S.C., Spence, R.R., Galvão, D.A & Newton, R.U. (2009) Australian Association for Exercise and Sport Science position stand: optimising cancer outcomes through exercise. *Journal of Science and Medicine in Sport, 12(4): 428-434.*

Holmes, M.D., Chen, W.Y., Feskanich, D., Kroenke, C.H. & Colditz, G.A. (2005). Physical activity and survival after breast cancer diagnosis. *Journal of the American Medical Association, 293: 2479-2486.*

Intercountry Adoption Australia. (2020). *Frequently Asked Questions.* Retrieved from https:www.intercountryadoption. gov.au

Irwin, M.L., Wilder Smith, A., McTiernan, A., et al. (2008). Influence of pre- and post-diagnosis physical activity on mortality in breast cancer survivors: The health, eating, activity, and lifestyle study. *Journal of Clinical Oncology, 26(24): 3958-3964.*

Lacomba, M.T., Sanchez, M.J.Y., Goni, A.I.Z. et al. (2010). Effectiveness of early physiotherapy to prevent lymphoedema after surgery for breast cancer: randomised, single-blinded, clinical trial. *British Medical Journal, 340: b5396.*

Lauridsen, M.C., Overgaard, M., Overgaard, J. et al. (2008). Shoulder disability and late symptoms following surgery for early breast cancer. *Acta Oncologica, 47(4): 569-575.*

McNeely, M.L., Binkley, J.M., Pusic, A.L., et al. (2012). A Prospective Model of Care for Breast Cancer Rehabilitation: Postoperative and Post-reconstructive Issues. *Cancer, 118 (8 suppl): 2226-2236.*

Moore, H.C.F., Unger, J.M., Phillips, K.A., et al. (2015). Goserelin for Ovarian Protection during Breast-Cancer Adjuvant Chemotherapy. *New England Journal of Medicine, 372(10): 923-932.*

National Breast Cancer Foundation Statistics (2020). Retrieved from https://nbcf.org.au/about-breast-cancer/breast-cancer-stats/

Ndlela, B., Sandhu, S., Lai, J. et al. (2018). Before, during, and after pregnancy cancer. *Journal of Global Oncology, 4, Supplement 2: 202s-202s.*

Olsson Möller, U., Beck, I., Rydén L. & Malmström, M. (2019). A comprehensive approach to rehabilitation interventions following breast cancer treatment – a systematic review of systematic reviews. *BioMed Central Cancer, 19: 472-492.*

References

Phillips, K.A., Collins, I.M., Milne R.L., et al. (2016). Anti-Müllerian hormone serum concentrations of women with germline BRCA1 or BRCA2 mutations. *Human Reproduction, 31(5): 1126–1132.*

Sample, I. (2007). *Women urged not to use frozen eggs as insurance.* Retrieved from https://www.theguardian.com/science/2007/oct/18/medicalresearch.health

Schadler, K.L., Thomas, N.J., Galie, P.A., et al. (2016). Tumor vessel normalization after aerobic exercise enhances chemotherapeutic efficacy. *Oncotarget, 7(40): 65429- 65440.*

Schmitz, K.H., Ahmed, R.L., Troxel, A.B. et al. (2010). Weight-Lifting for Women at Risk for Breast Cancer–Related Lymphedema. *Journal of the American Medical Association, 304(24): 2699-2705.*

Smith, S. (2014). Functional morbidity following latissimus dorsi flap breast reconstruction. *Journal of the Advanced Practitioner in Oncology, 5(3): 181–187.*

Sowa, Y., Morihara, T., Kushida R., et al. (2016). Long-term prospective assessment of shoulder function after breast reconstruction involving a latissimus dorsi muscle flap transfer and postoperative radiotherapy. *Breast Cancer, 24(3): 362-368.*

Stan, D.L., Rausch, S.M., Sundt, K., et al. (2012). Pilates for breast cancer survivors. *Clinical Journal of Oncology Nursing, 16(2): 131-41.*

Stuiver M.M., ten Tusscher M.R., Agasi-Idenburg C.S. et al. (2015). *Conservative interventions for preventing clinically detectable upper-limb lymphoedema in patients who are at risk of developing lymphoedema after breast cancer therapy (Review).* The Cochrane Collaboration: John Wiley & Sons, Ltd. Issue 2.

Suami, H., Heydon-White, A., Mackie, H. et al. (2019). A new indocyanine green fluorescence lymphography protocol for identification of the lymphatic drainage pathway for patients with breast cancer-related lymphoedema. *BioMed Central Cancer,* 19: 985-991.

Taschery, S. (2014). *Inflammation and cancer: Why your diet is important.* Retrieved from https://www.mdanderson.org/publications/focused-on-health/inflamation-cancer-diet

Yilmaz M., Elmali A., Yazici, G. (2019) Abscopal Effect, From Myth to Reality: From Radiation Oncologist's Perspective. *Cureus 11(1): e3860.*

About the Author

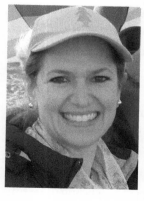

Petrina graduated from Curtin University, Perth, in 1996 with a Bachelor of Science of Physiotherapy, and has worked in various clinical areas in both Australia and abroad. Upon turning 30, she asked her medical practitioners about her cancer risk due to the breast and ovarian cancers on her father's side of the family, only to be diagnosed soon afterward at 31 with an aggressive form of breast cancer. Petrina discovered a year later that she carried the BRCA1 gene mutation, also carried by her father, aunt, cousin and grandmother.

Having personally experienced the gap in allied health service provisions in oncology, Petrina established a comprehensive and innovative rehabilitation and wellness service called Breast, Gynae, and Lymph Physiotherapy in Perth, Western Australia, in

2009. Over the 12 years since it was established, she has brought a unique specialist skillset from her qualifications, combined with her in-depth personal understanding of cancer recovery, to specifically provide management and rehabilitation of breast and gynaecologic cancer and lymphoedema. Now at 14 years post-diagnosis, Petrina and her allied health team have helped many women (and men) by providing holistic cancer physiotherapy and rehabilitation, dietetics and exercise physiology services.

As a sessional lecturer in oncology, Petrina has enjoyed teaching Curtin University post-graduate and Notre Dame undergraduate physiotherapy students. In addition to her professional work, Petrina has also been an active consumer representative, advocating for cancer consumers for various government, research, and not-for-profit charities, including the Breast Cancer Network Australia, Breast Cancer Trials Australia, Cancer Australia and Medicare.

Now in 2021, after having personally treated over 2000 people with cancer, Petrina is providing clinical leadership and support to BGAL, having stepped back from direct patient consultation. She continues to use her skills and passions in cancer care advocacy and allied health management. She is enjoying spending more time with her "man" and fox terrier dogs at Perth's glorious beaches and the Western Australian outdoors.

Petrina Burnett
M.B.A. (Leadership & Innovation), M. Clinical. Physiotherapy (Continence & Women's Health)
B. Science (Physiotherapy), Dip. Pilates (Polestar Rehabilitation).
Level 2 Lymphoedema Practitioner.

Acknowledgements

—•—

I would like to gratefully acknowledge the stedfast support and assistance of many people and organisations, including;

Dr. Linley Mitchell, Dr. David Ingram, Prof. Arlene Chan, Dr. Mandy Taylor, Dr. Albert Tiong, Dr. Jenny Slee, Dr. Lucy Williams, Dr. Chris Finn, Dr. Stuart Salfinger, Assoc. Prof. Paul Cohen, Dr. Peter Willsher, Dr. Tony Connell, Dr. Marcus Chin, Prof. Christobel Saunders, Dr. Lee Jackson, Dr. Wen Chan Yeow, Dr. Tim Clay, Ms Cynthia Edgerton-Warburton, Dr. Adeline Fong, The Fong Family, Dr. Lesley Ramage, Ms. Joan Burgess, Ms. Gay Refeld, Dr. Pam Hendry, Ms. Leanne Taylor, Ms. Fiona Hancock, Ms. Christine Jones, Ms. Cath Griffiths, Ms. Sheryl Potts, Ms. Sarah Ang, Ms. Julie Richmond, Ms. Vanessa Cooke, Ms. Jenny Pope, Ms. Rachel Bootsma, Ms. Jenny Grant, Assoc. Prof Kathy Briffa, Ms. Lynn Swinburne, Ms. Kirsten Pilatti, Ms. Amanda Winiata, Ms. Kathy Wells, Ms. Lisa Morstyn, Dr. Soozy Smith, Ms. Anna Fitzgerald, Ms. Julie Callaghan, Ms. Amanda Bott, Ms. Lisa-Maree Ellett, Ms. Pilsy Corbo, Ms. Nicki Doyle, Ms. Ryah Eastman, Mr. Ken and Ms.

Shirley Friday, Mr. John Browne, Ms. Jo Marwick, Ms. Rebecca Lewis, Ms. Veronica Acuna, Ms. Jo Morris, Ms. Berit Jardine, Ms. Tania Ciavalini, Ms. Jesse Chandler, Ms. Loretta Bird, Mr. David Wickham, Ms. Patricia Price, Ms. Molly McGurk, Ms. Annabelle Kubo, Ms. Evelin Kubo, Ms. Anita Johnson, Ms. Toni Johnson, Ms. Leah Blinkhorn, Ms. Katja Webb, Dr. Jill Sullivan, Ms. Triona Walsh, Ms. Marilyn Arkeveld, Ms. Vicki McKenzie, Mr. Cameron Harris, Ms. Libby Hargreaves, Ms. Joe Wiggett, Ms. Jude Tozer, Ms. Alysia Kepert, Ms. Tanya Sim, Ms. Tracey Lewis, Ms. Tracey Taggart, Ms. Anne-Marie D'Arcy, Ms. Susannah Morris, Ms. Leonie Young, Ms. Leslie Gilham, Ms. Patricia Hancock, Ms. Libby Burgess, Ms. Sandi Stanford, Ms. Dale Eastman, Ms. Judith Gedalia, Ms. Denise Barlow, The Mount Hospital, Sir Charles Gairdner Hospital, King Edward Memorial Hospital, St John of God Hospital Subiaco, Perth Radiological Clinic, Pathology Services in WA, Claremont Medical, Divas and Divos for Cancer team, Breast Cancer Network Australia, Breast Cancer Care WA, Solaris Cancer Care, Breast Cancer Trials Australia, BINGWA Nursing Group, Alamo Breast Cancer Foundation, National Breast Cancer Coalition, Pink Hope, Ovarian Cancer Australia, friends and supporters of BGAL Physiotherapy, numerous nursing, care and theatre staff and many many others.

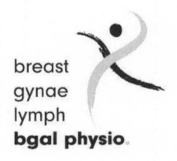

breast
gynae
lymph
bgal physio

BGAL Physiotherapy is a leading oncology allied health practice committed to clinical excellence, located in Perth, Western Australia. Founded in 2009 by Petrina Burnett, the practice provides holistic, comprehensive, individualised and evidence-based cancer care. Services include both clinic-based and telehealth consultations in breast & gynae oncology physiotherapy services, lymphoedema care, exercise physiology/ physiotherapy and dietetics care. Rebates may be accessed through Australian Private Health Insurance, Medicare Australia, Veterans Affairs and Workcover. Referrals are not required if using Australian Private Health Insurance or if self funded.

Address: Unit 1, 21 Roydhouse St
Subiaco 6008
Perth, Western Australia
Ph: (+61) 08 6162 2964
Email: admin@bgalphysio.com.au
Website: www.bgalphysio.com.au

Cancer Organisation Contact Details

•────────────────────•

Breast Cancer Network Australia- information, advocacy, networking, and support.

293 Camberwell Rd
Camberwell, VIC 3124
Ph: 1800 260 243
contact@bcna.org.au
www.bcna.org.au

Breast Cancer Care Western Australia- support, networking, and information.
80 Railway Street, Cottesloe WA 6011
info@breastcancer.org.au
Ph:(08) 9324 3703

Pink Hope- information for high-risk breast cancer.
PO Box 725, Narrabeen NSW 2101
Ph: 02 8084 2288
info@pinkhope.org.au
www.pinkhope.org.au

Reclaim Your Curves- support, inform, and network around breast reconstruction.
admin@reclaimyourcurves.org.au
www.reclaimyourcurves.org.au

Cancer Council Australia- support, inform, and fund cancer research.
Tel: (02) 8063 4100
info@cancer.org.au
www.cancer.org.au

Cancer Australia- establish Australian national clinical guidelines.
Postal address: Locked Bag 3, STRAWBERRY HILLS NSW 2012
Ph: +61 2 9357 9400 or 1800 624 973
enquiries@canceraustralia.gov.au
https://www.canceraustralia.gov.au/

Solaris Cancer Care, Western Australia- provides complementary and integrated medicines.
80 Railway Street
Cottesloe, WA 6011
Ph: (08) 9384 3544
www.solariscancercare.org.au

Ovarian Cancer Australia- advocate, network, inform, and support.
Level 1, 210 Lonsdale St, Melbourne, VIC 3000
tel:1300-660-334
support@ovariancancer.net.au
www.ovariancancer.net.au

Breast Cancer Trials Australia & New Zealand- research, science, and advocacy training for consumers.
PO Box 283
The Junction NSW 2291
Australia
tel: 1800 423 444
www.breastcancertrials.org.au

Ovarian Cancer Research Foundation- fund research
PO Box 428, Ashburton, Victoria 3147
Ph: 1300 682 742
community@ocrf.com.au
www.ocrf.com.au

The Ladybird Foundation (fund West Australian Breast and Gynae Cancer Research)
www.ladybirdfoundation.org.au

National Breast Cancer Coalition- advocate, inform, network
1010 Vermont Ave, NW, Suite 900
Washington DC 20005 USA
Ph: 800-622-2838
info@stopbreastcancer.org
www.stopbreastcancer.org

Alamo Breast Cancer Foundation- breast science and advocacy training for consumers- national and international.
PO Box 780067 San Antonio Texas 78278-0067
info@alamobreastcancer.org
https://www.alamobreastcancer.org/

Young Survival Coalition- support, advocate, inform, network.
75 Broad St, Suite 409
New York, NY 10004
Ph: 877.972.1011
www.youngsurvival.org

Australian Lymphology Association- information, connect with health professionals
PO Box 7345, Beaumaris, VIC 3193
Ph: 1300 935 332
admin@lymphoedema.org.au
https://www.lymphoedema.org.au/

Australian Physiotherapy Association Cancer, Palliative Care and Lymphoedema Group- professional body for physiotherapists
Ph: +61 3 9092 0888
info@australian.physio
www.australian.physio/membership/national-groups/cancer-palliative-care-and-lymphoedema

Lightning Source UK Ltd.
Milton Keynes UK
UKHW010940270722
406450UK00002B/368